Haematology and
the Asian Patient

Haematology encompasses a broad range of topics ranging from common and relatively benign conditions such as iron deficiency anaemia and hereditary diseases such as thalassaemia, to haematological malignancies that are often life-threatening. Burgeoning information arising from technological advances in recent years has made these subjects particularly challenging for medical students and non-specialist medical practitioners. This book aims to highlight the pathophysiology, clinical presentations and basic principles in the investigation and management of haematological diseases that are prevalent in Asia. Each chapter begins with a real-case clinical scenario, followed by a set of questions, and is complemented by photomicrographs, data charts and illustrations. Readers will have a basic knowledge in haematology, and the book will be a useful reference in their academic study and clinical encounters.

T0321059

Haematology and the Asian Patient
51 Clinical Cases

Anskar Y.H. Leung
Edmond S.K. Ma

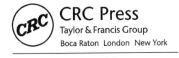

CRC Press
Taylor & Francis Group
Boca Raton London New York

CRC Press is an imprint of the
Taylor & Francis Group, an **informa** business

Designed cover image: Authors

First edition published 2024
by CRC Press
2385 NW Executive Center Drive, Suite 320, Boca Raton FL 33431

and by CRC Press
4 Park Square, Milton Park, Abingdon, Oxon, OX14 4RN

CRC Press is an imprint of Taylor & Francis Group, LLC

Library of Congress Cataloging-in-Publication Data
Names: Leung, Anskar Y. H. (Anskar Yu-Hung), author. ǀ Ma, Edmond S. K. (Edmond Shui Kwan), author.
Title: Haematology and the Asian patient : 51 clinical cases / Anskar Y.H. Leung, Edmond S.K. Ma.
Description: First edition. ǀ Boca Raton, FL : CRC Press, 2024. ǀ Includes bibliographical references and index.
Identifiers: LCCN 2024009965 (print) ǀ LCCN 2024009966 (ebook) ǀ ISBN 9781032351261 (hardback) ǀ
    ISBN 9781032351254 (paperback) ǀ ISBN 9781003325413 (ebook)
Subjects: MESH: Hematologic Diseases—epidemiology ǀ Hematologic Diseases—physiopathology ǀ
    Hematologic Diseases—therapy ǀ Asian People ǀ Asia—epidemiology ǀ Case Reports
Classification: LCC RC636 (print) ǀ LCC RC636 (ebook) ǀ NLM WH 120 ǀ DDC 616.1/50089914—dc23/eng/20240405
LC record available at https://lccn.loc.gov/2024009965
LC ebook record available at https://lccn.loc.gov/2024009966

ISBN: 978-1-032-35126-1 (hbk)
ISBN: 978-1-032-35125-4 (pbk)
ISBN: 978-1-003-32541-3 (ebk)

DOI: 10.1201/9781003325413

Typeset in Times LT Std
by Apex CoVantage, LLC

Contents

Foreword I xix
Foreword II xxi
About the Authors xxiii
Acknowledgements xxv

Haemostasis and Thrombosis

Chapter 1   Von Willebrand Disease 3

    1.1 Clinical Scenario 3
    1.2 Laboratory Reports 3
    1.3 Questions 3
    1.4 Clinical Progress 3
    1.5 Von Willebrand Factor (VWF) 4
    1.6 Von Willebrand Disease (VWD) 4
    1.7 Diagnosis 5
    1.8 Differential Diagnosis 5
    1.9 Management 5
    1.10 Key Points 6
    Additional Readings 6

Chapter 2   Severe Haemophilia 7

    2.1 Clinical Scenario 7
    2.2 Laboratory Reports 7
    2.3 Questions 7
    2.4 Haemophilia A 7
    2.5 Genetics 7
    2.6 Genetic Testing 8
    2.7 Differential Diagnosis 9
    2.8 Management 9
    2.9 Key Points 10
    Additional Readings 10

Chapter 3   Factor VII Deficiency 11

    3.1 Clinical Scenario 11
    3.2 Laboratory Reports 11
    3.3 Questions 11
    3.4 Progress 11
        3.4.1 Factor VII 11
        3.4.2 Factor VII Deficiency 12
    3.5 Clinical Presentation 12
    3.6 Treatment 13
    3.7 Differential Diagnosis 13

3.8   Key Points... 13
Additional Reading 13

Chapter 4 Acquired Haemophilia 14

4.1   Clinical Scenario... 14
4.2   Laboratory Reports... 14
4.3   Questions 14
4.4   Clinical Progress 14
4.5   Isolated APTT Prolongation.. 14
4.6   Laboratory Confirmation of Acquired Factor VIII Inhibitor........................ 16
4.7   Causes of Acquired Factor VIII Inhibitor... 16
4.8   Treatment.. 16
4.9   Key Points... 17
Additional Reading 17

Chapter 5 Acquired Factor V Inhibitor 18

5.1   Clinical Scenario... 18
5.2   Laboratory Reports... 18
5.3   Questions 18
5.4   Clinical Progress 18
5.5   Interpretation of Prolonged PT and APTT.. 18
5.5.1   Acquired Factor V Inhibitor.. 19
5.6   Key Points... 20
Additional Reading 20

Chapter 6 Disseminated Intravascular Coagulopathy 21

6.1   Clinical Scenario... 21
6.2   Laboratory Reports... 21
6.3   Questions 21
6.4   Diagnosis 21
6.5   Pathogenesis 22
6.6   Management of DIC 23
6.7   Key Points... 23
Additional Readings.. 23

Chapter 7 Cancer-Related Thrombosis 24

7.1   Clinical Scenario... 24
7.2   Laboratory Reports... 24
7.3   Questions 24
7.4   Clinical Progress 24
7.5   Pathogenesis 24
7.6   Risk Factors of VTE... 25
7.7   Diagnosis of VTE... 27
7.8   Treatment.. 27
7.9   Duration of Treatment 28
7.10   Complications of VTE.. 28
7.11   Key Points... 28
Additional Reading 28

Myeloid Malignancy

Chapter 8 Acute Myeloid Leukaemia I..31

    8.1 Clinical Scenario 31
    8.2 Laboratory Reports...31
    8.3 Questions 31
    8.4 Clinical Progress 31
    8.5 Acute Myeloid Leukaemia—Diagnosis 32
    8.6 Clinical Presentation 33
    8.7 Prognostication 33
    8.8 MRD Monitoring..33
    8.9 Management of AML 33
    8.10 Key Points..34
    Additional Reading 34

Chapter 9 Acute Myeloid Leukaemia II 35

    9.1 Clinical Scenario 35
    9.2 Laboratory Reports...35
    9.3 Questions 35
    9.4 Patient Progress 35
    9.5 Acute Myeloid Leukaemia (AML) 35
    9.6 Treatment of Acute Myeloid Leukaemia in the Elderly 37
    9.7 BCL2 Inhibitor 37
    9.8 Key Points..37
    Additional Readings 38

Chapter 10 Myelodysplastic Syndrome 39

    10.1 Clinical Scenario 39
    10.2 Laboratory Reports...39
    10.3 Questions 39
    10.4 Progress 39
    10.5 Further Question...39
    10.6 Progress 40
    10.7 Myelodysplastic Syndrome...40
    10.8 Pathogenesis 41
    10.9 Differential Diagnosis 41
    10.10 Treatment...41
    10.11 Key Points..42
    Additional Reading 42

Chapter 11 Chronic Myeloid Leukaemia..43

    11.1 Clinical Scenario 43
    11.2 Laboratory Reports...43
    11.3 Questions 43
    11.4 Clinical Progress 43
    11.5 Pathogenesis 43
    11.6 Clinical Presentation 44
    11.7 Laboratory Diagnosis 46

11.8 Prognostic Factors 46
11.9 Natural Disease Course 46
11.10 Management of CML 46
11.11 Monitoring Treatment Response to TKI 46
11.12 Key Points 47
Additional Reading 47

Chapter 12 Essential Thrombocytosis 48
12.1 Clinical Scenario 48
12.2 Laboratory Reports 48
12.3 Questions 48
12.4 Clinical Progress 48
12.5 Differential Diagnosis and Clinical Presentation 48
12.6 Genetics of Essential Thrombocytosis 49
12.7 Complications of Essential Thrombocytosis 50
12.8 Prognosis 50
12.9 Treatment 50
12.10 Key Points 50
Additional Readings 50

Chapter 13 Polycythaemia Vera 51
13.1 Clinical Scenario 51
13.2 Laboratory Reports in 2013 51
13.3 Questions 51
13.4 Clinical Progress 51
13.5 Laboratory Reports in 2021 51
13.6 Clinical Features 52
13.7 Prognosis 53
13.8 Complications 53
13.9 Management Plan 53
13.10 Key Points 53
Additional Reading 53

Chapter 14 Primary Myelofibrosis 54
14.1 Clinical Scenario 54
14.2 Laboratory Reports 54
14.3 Questions 54
14.4 Clinical Progress 54
14.5 Clinical Presentation 54
14.6 Diagnosis 55
14.7 Prognostication 56
14.8 Treatment 56
14.9 Key Points 56
Additional Reading 57

Chapter 15 Myeloid Neoplasm with Germline Predisposition 58
15.1 Clinical Scenario 58
15.2 Investigations and Patient Progress 58

15.3 Questions 58
15.4 Patient Progress 58
15.5 Myeloid Neoplasm with Germline Predisposition 58
15.6 Myeloid Neoplasms with Germline *RUNX1* Mutation 60
15.7 Key Points 60
Additional Reading 60

Chapter 16 Langerhans Cell Histiocytosis 61
16.1 Clinical Scenario 61
16.2 Questions 61
16.3 Langerhans Cell Histiocytosis 61
16.4 Other Histiocytosis 64
16.5 Key Points 64
Additional Readings 64

Lymphoid Malignancy

Chapter 17 Diffuse Large B-Cell Lymphoma 67
17.1 Clinical Scenario 67
17.2 Diffuse Large B-Cell Lymphoma—Overview 67
17.3 Aetiology 67
17.4 Cell of Origin 69
17.5 Molecular Landscape 69
17.6 Clinical Presentation 69
17.7 Management 69
17.8 Prognostication 70
17.9 Key Points 70
Additional Readings 70

Chapter 18 Waldenström Macroglobulinaemia 71
18.1 Clinical Scenario 71
18.2 Laboratory Reports 71
18.3 Questions 71
18.4 Clinical Progress 71
18.5 Waldenström Macroglobulinaemia 71
18.6 Clinical Manifestations 72
18.7 Diagnosis 73
    18.7.1 Management of Waldenström Macroglobulinaemia 73
18.8 Key Points 73
Additional Readings 74

Chapter 19 Chronic Lymphocytic Leukaemia 75
19.1 Clinical Scenario 75
19.2 Laboratory Reports 75
19.3 Questions 75
19.4 Clinical Progress 75

19.5   Chronic Lymphocytic Leukaemia...77
19.6   Diagnosis...77
19.7   Prognostication..77
19.8   Principle of Management 78
19.9   Key Points...78
Additional Readings..79

Chapter 20   Hairy Cell Leukaemia 80
20.1   Clinical Scenario...80
20.2   Laboratory Reports..80
20.3   Questions...80
20.4   Clinical Progress 80
20.5   Hairy Cell Leukaemia 81
20.6   HCL Variant 82
20.7   Key Points...82
Additional Reading 82

Chapter 21   Philadelphia Chromosome–Positive Acute Lymphoblastic Leukaemia.....................83
21.1   Clinical Scenario...83
21.2   Laboratory Reports..83
21.3   Questions...83
21.4   Patient Progress 83
21.5   Precursor B-Cell ALL 85
21.6   Philadelphia Chromosome–Positive ALL...85
21.7   Treatment of Ph+ ALL 85
21.8   Key Points...86
Additional Readings..86

Chapter 22   Natural Killer Cell Lymphoma..87
22.1   Clinical Scenario...87
22.2   Questions...87
22.3   Clinical Progress 87
22.4   NK/T-Cell Lymphoma 87
22.5   Clinical Subtypes of NK/T-Cell Lymphoma 87
22.6   Key Points...89
Additional Reading 89

Chapter 23   Mycosis Fungoides..90
23.1   Clinical Scenario...90
23.2   Questions...90
23.3   Mycosis Fungoides 90
23.4   Clinical Presentation 90
23.5   Staging of Mycosis Fungoides..90
23.6   Key Points...92
Additional Readings..92

Chapter 24 T-cell Prolymphocytic Leukaemia 93

    24.1   Clinical Scenario 93
    24.2   Laboratory Reports..93
    24.3   Questions 93
    24.4   Clinical Progress 93
    24.5   T-PLL..94
    24.6   Management 94
    24.7   Key Points..95
    Additional Reading 95

Chapter 25 Hodgkin Lymphoma...96

    25.1   Clinical Scenario 96
    25.2   Questions 96
    25.3   Clinical Progress 96
    25.4   Differential Diagnoses...98
    25.5   Treatment and Prognosis 98
    25.6   Key Points..99
    Additional Reading 99

Plasma Cell Neoplasms

Chapter 26 Amyloidosis 103

    26.1   Clinical Scenario 103
    26.2   Laboratory Reports..103
    26.3   Questions 103
    26.4   Diagnosis 103
    26.5   Amyloidosis 105
    26.6   Clinical Presentation 105
    26.7   Investigations..105
    26.8   Management 106
    26.9   Key Points..106
    Additional Reading 106

Chapter 27 Multiple Myeloma...107

    27.1   Clinical Scenario 107
    27.2   Laboratory Reports..107
    27.3   Questions 107
    27.4   Progress 107
    27.5   Treatment Progress 108
    27.6   Multiple Myeloma..109
    27.7   Pathogenesis 110
    27.8   Clinical Features...110
    27.9   Investigations..110

27.10   Prognostication 110
27.11   Management Approach 111
27.12   Key Points 112
Additional Readings 112

Chapter 28 POEMS Syndrome 113

28.1   Clinical Scenario 113
28.2   Laboratory Reports 113
28.3   Questions 113
28.4   POEMS Syndrome 113
28.5   Patient Progress 115
28.6   Treatment 116
28.7   Key Points 116
Additional Reading 116

Thalassaemia and Haemoglobin Disorders

Chapter 29 Beta Thalassaemia Major 119

29.1   Clinical Scenario 119
29.2   Laboratory Reports 119
29.3   Questions 119
29.4   Clinical Progress 119
29.5   Beta Thalassaemia 120
29.6   Complications 121
29.7   Management 122
29.8   Key Points 122
Additional Readings 122

Chapter 30 Haemoglobin H Disease 123

30.1   Clinical Scenario 123
30.2   Laboratory Reports at Presentation 123
30.3   Questions 123
30.4   Clinical Progress 123
30.5   Thalassaemia Syndromes 124
30.6   Pathogenesis of Haemoglobin H Disease 124
30.7   Clinical Presentations 125
30.8   Laboratory Findings 125
30.9   Differential Diagnosis 125
30.10   Management 126
30.11   Key Points 126
Additional Readings 126

Chapter 31 Sickle Cell Disease 127

31.1   Clinical Scenario 127
31.2   Laboratory Reports 127
31.3   Questions 127

31.4   Clinical Progress 127
31.5   Sickle Cell Disease 129
31.6   Pathogenesis 129
31.7   Management 129
31.8   Prevention of Sickling Crises 129
31.9   Acute Sickling Crises and their Management 129
31.10   Chronic Sickle Cell Diseases and their Management 130
31.11   Key Points.. 130
         Additional Reading 130

Chapter 32 Methaemoglobinaemia 131
32.1   Clinical Scenario 131
32.2   Laboratory Reports.. 131
32.3   Questions 131
32.4   Clinical Progress 131
32.5   Laboratory Reports.. 131
32.6   Normal Oxygen Transfer in Haemoglobin 132
32.7   Drawback of Pulse Oximetry in Methaemoglobinaemia....... 133
32.8   Saturation Gap.. 133
32.9   Causes of Methaemoglobinaemia....................................... 133
32.10   Clinical Presentation 133
32.11   Treatment... 134
32.12   Key Points.. 134
         Additional Reading 134

Nutritional and Aplastic Anaemia

Chapter 33 Aplastic Anaemia 137
33.1   Clinical Scenario.. 137
33.2   Laboratory Reports.. 137
33.3   Questions 137
33.4   Investigations... 137
33.5   Clinical Progress 138
33.6   Aplastic Anaemia 139
33.7   Pathophysiology.. 139
33.8   Differential Diagnosis 139
33.9   Management Approach... 140
33.10   Key Points.. 140
         Additional Readings.. 140

Chapter 34 Iron Deficiency Anaemia... 141
34.1   Clinical Scenario 141
34.2   Laboratory Results 141
34.3   Questions 141
34.4   Iron Metabolism 141
34.5   Causes.. 143

34.6   Symptoms 143
34.7   Investigations 143
34.8   Treatment 144
34.9   Key Points 144
Additional Readings 144

Chapter 35 Vitamin B12 Deficiency Anaemia 145
35.1   Clinical Scenario 145
35.2   Laboratory Reports 145
35.3   Questions 145
35.4   Clinical Progress 145
35.5   Further Laboratory Tests 145
35.6   Sources of Vitamin B12 in the Body 146
35.7   Dietary Vitamin B12 Absorption 147
35.8   Cellular Function of Vitamin B12 147
35.9   Clinical Manifestations 147
35.10   Laboratory Features 147
35.11   Bone Marrow Features 148
35.12   Causes 148
35.13   Pernicious Anaemia 148
35.14   Treatment 149
35.15   Key Points 149
Additional Reading 149

Haemolytic Anaemia

Chapter 36 Warm-Type Autoimmune Haemolytic Anaemia 153
36.1   Clinical Scenario 153
36.2   Laboratory Reports 153
36.3   Questions 153
36.4   Diagnosis 153
36.5   Pathogenesis 154
36.6   Differential Diagnosis 154
36.7   Management 155
36.8   Key Points 155
Additional Readings 155

Chapter 37 Cold Agglutinin Disease 156
37.1   Clinical Scenario 156
37.2   Laboratory Reports 156
37.3   Questions 156
37.4   Clinical Progress 156
37.5   Cold Agglutinin Disease 156
37.6   Pathogenesis of Haemolysis in CAD 157
37.7   Cold Agglutinin Syndrome 158
37.8   Investigations 158

37.9   Treatment...158
37.10   Key Points...158
Additional Readings...158

Chapter 38 G6PD Deficiency..159
38.1   Clinical Scenario..159
38.2   Laboratory Reports...159
38.3   Questions...159
38.4   Clinical Progress...159
38.5   G6PD Physiology...159
38.6   Genetics...160
38.7   Haematological Effects...161
38.8   Diagnosis...161
38.9   Management..162
38.10   Key Points...162
Additional Readings...162

Chapter 39 Hereditary Spherocytosis..163
39.1   Clinical Scenario..163
39.2   Laboratory Reports...163
39.3   Questions...163
39.4   Hereditary Spherocytosis...163
39.5   Diagnosis...164
39.6   Genetic Basis...165
39.7   Management..165
39.8   Key Points...165
Additional Readings...165

Chapter 40 Paravalvular Leak...166
40.1   Clinical Scenario...166
40.2   Laboratory Reports..166
40.3   Questions..166
40.4   Clinical Progress..166
40.5   Cardiac Prosthesis-Related Haemolytic Anaemia 167
40.6   Key Points..167
Additional Reading 168

Chapter 41 Paroxysmal Nocturnal Haemoglobinuria.........................169
41.1   Clinical Scenario...169
41.2   Laboratory Reports..169
41.3   Questions..169
41.4   Clinical Progress..169
41.5   Pathogenesis...170
41.6   Clinical Manifestations 171
41.7   Diagnosis..171
41.8   Treatment...171
41.9   Key Points..172
Additional Readings...172

Chapter 42 Thrombotic Thrombocytopenic Purpura 173

    42.1   Clinical Scenario.. 173

    42.2   Laboratory Reports.. 173

    42.3   Questions 173

    42.4   Clinical Progress 173

    42.5   Differential Diagnosis of Thrombotic Microangiopathy 175

    42.6   Pathogenesis 175

    42.7   Clinical Features.. 175

    42.8   Causes.. 175

    42.9   Investigations 176

    42.10   Management Approach.. 176

    42.11   Key Points... 176

    Additional Readings 176

Chapter 43 Atypical Haemolytic Uraemic Syndrome 177

    43.1   Clinical Scenario.. 177

    43.2   Laboratory Reports.. 177

           43.2.1   Haematology 177

           43.2.2   Biochemistry 177

    43.3   Questions 177

    43.4   Clinical Progress 178

    43.5   Thrombotic Microangiopathy During Pregnancy....................... 178

    43.6   Haemolytic Uraemic Syndrome.. 178

    43.7   Classification 179

    43.8   Diagnosis 179

    43.9   Management 179

    43.10   Key Points... 180

    Additional Reading 180

Thrombocytopenia

Chapter 44 Immune Thrombocytopenia 183

    44.1   Clinical Scenario.. 183

    44.2   Laboratory Reports.. 183

    44.3   Questions 183

    44.4   Clinical Progress 183

    44.5   Clinical Features.. 183

    44.6   Pathogenesis 184

    44.7   Diagnosis 185

    44.8   Management 185

    44.9   Key Points... 186

    Additional Readings 186

Chapter 45 Hereditary Macrothrombocytopenia 187

    45.1   Clinical Scenario.. 187

    45.2   Laboratory Reports.. 187

45.3   Questions 187
45.4   Clinical Progress 187
45.5   Hereditary Macrothrombocytopenia—Clinical Spectrum 187
45.6   Diagnosis 189
45.7   Clinical Relevance 189
45.8   Key Points 189
Additional Readings 189

Miscellaneous Conditions

Chapter 46 Castleman Disease 193

46.1   Clinical Scenario 193
46.2   Laboratory Reports 193
46.3   Questions 193
46.4   Clinical Progress 193
46.5   Castleman Disease 193
46.6   Diagnosis 195
46.7   Management 195
46.8   Key Points 195
Additional Readings 195

Chapter 47 Haemophagocytic Lymphohistiocytosis 196

47.1   Clinical Scenario 196
47.2   Laboratory Reports 196
        47.2.1 Haematology 196
        47.2.2 Biochemistry 196
47.3   Clinical Progress 196
47.4   Questions 197
47.5   Diagnosis 198
47.6   Pathophysiology 198
47.7   Clinical Presentation 198
47.8   Diagnosis 198
47.9   Treatment 199
47.10   Key Points 199
Additional Readings 199

Chapter 48 Hypereosinophilia 200

48.1   Clinical Scenario 200
48.2   Laboratory Reports 200
48.3   Questions 200
48.4   Clinical Progress 200
48.5   Eosinophilia 201
48.6   Hypereosinophilic Syndrome 202
48.7   Clinical Presentation 202
48.8   Management 202
48.9   Key Points 203
Additional Readings 203

Chapter 49 IgG4–Related Disease 204

    49.1   Clinical Scenario 204
    49.2   Laboratory Reports...204
    49.3   Questions 204
    49.4   IgG4–Related Disease 204
    49.5   Investigations...205
    49.6   Differential Diagnoses..206
    49.7   Treatment...206
    49.8   Key Points..206
    Additional Reading 206

Chapter 50 Lymphadenopathy and Hypergammaglobulinaemia...............................207

    50.1   Clinical Scenario 207
    50.2   Laboratory Reports...207
    50.3   Questions 207
    50.4   Causes...207
    50.5   Investigations...209
    50.6   Clinical Progress 209
    50.7   Human Immunodeficiency Virus (HIV) Infection...........................209
    50.8   Key Points..209
    Additional Reading 209

Chapter 51 Paraneoplastic Pemphigus..210

    51.1   Clinical Scenario 210
    51.2   Laboratory Reports...210
    51.3   Questions 210
    51.4   Clinical Progress 210
    51.5   Paraneoplastic Pemphigus...212
    51.6   Pathogenesis 212
    51.7   Treatment...212
    51.8   Key Points..213
    Additional Readings 213

Index..215

Foreword I

Clinical haematology is a wonderfully diverse subject as it spans both laboratory diagnosis and patient management. Rapid advances in genomics and molecular biology, together with the development of novel therapeutics, many of which have dramatically improved patient outcomes, have made haematology a fascinating subject for trainees and specialists alike. However, for medical students and non-specialists, the breadth of haematology can be overwhelming, particularly during their preparation for examinations. This book by Prof. Anskar Y.H. Leung and Dr. Edmond S.K. Ma, seasoned examiners in clinical and laboratory haematology in Hong Kong, provides a practical account of 51 haematology cases that cover topics ranging from "benign" and consultation haematology to haematological malignancies, including diseases that are prevalent in Asia. I am particularly fond of the case-based approach that is complemented by illustrations, analysis of treatment outcomes and excellent photographs, whose combination makes this not only a handy book for undergraduate and MRCP examination preparation but also a quick look-up reference during clinical practice. It focuses on principles and covers areas where recent advances, particularly in haematological malignancies, have improved diagnostics and/or management.

I congratulate both authors on this book and hope readers will find this case-based approach as enjoyable and informative as I did when I was training.

Professor A.R. Green PhD, FRCP, FRCPath, FMedSci
Emeritus Professor of Haemato-Oncology
Wellcome-MRC Cambridge Stem Cell Institute and Department of Haematology
University of Cambridge

Foreword II

For medical students and non-specialists, clinical haematology is a broad discipline and many haematologic diseases involve complex processes that are often difficult to understand. This is complicated by the rapidly emerging information about the genetics and molecular biology of blood diseases and the advent of novel therapeutics. This book by Prof. Anskar Y.H. Leung and Dr. Edmond S.K. Ma, both experienced examiners for undergraduate students and postgraduate fellows in Hong Kong, will be a comprehensive source of information covering a wide range of haematologic diseases, many of which are prevalent in Asia. Each topic begins with a real clinical scenario and laboratory reports, followed by a succinct description of pathogenetic mechanisms and the treatment outcome for each scenario. The book is easy to read and contains illustrations of disease pathogeneses and photomicrographs of cell morphology. I found the treatment outcome of each scenario particularly impressive, and it underscored the impact of novel therapeutics on patient outcomes.

I offer my heartfelt congratulations to these authors on producing a book that will be a very useful reference for doctors in Asia in their preparation of examinations and management of haematologic diseases.

Mark James Levis, MD, PhD
Professor of Oncology
Program Leader, Haematologic Malignancies and Bone Marrow Transplant Program
Sidney Kimmel Comprehensive Cancer Center
Johns Hopkins University

About the Authors

Prof. Anskar Y.H. Leung is currently Chair Professor of Haematology and Deputy Chairperson in the Department of Medicine at the University of Hong Kong (HKU). He graduated with an MBChB (Hons) and PhD from the Chinese University of Hong Kong (CUHK) in 1996 and joined HKU as Clinical Assistant Professor in 1999. He earned his specialist qualification in haematology and haematological oncology in 2003 and was promoted to Clinical Associate Professor and Clinical Professor in 2007 and 2012, respectively.

Dr. Edmond S.K. Ma earned his MBBS and MD degrees from HKU in 1987 and 2004. He is currently the Director of Clinical and Molecular Pathology at the Hong Kong Sanatorium and Hospital, Honorary Clinical Associate Professor at the Department of Pathology HKU, and Clinical Associate Professor (Honorary) at the Department of Anatomical and Cellular Pathology CUHK. He was previously Vice-President and Chief Examiner in Haematology at the Hong Kong College of Pathologists and is past Chairman of the Hong Kong Society for the Study of Thalassaemia and Hong Kong Association of Blood Transfusion and Haematology. He is currently Chairman of the Children's Thalassaemia Foundation.

Acknowledgements

The authors wanted to thank Mr. Keith Fung and Ms. Winki Lai who have contributed substantially to the creation of illustrations and manuscript editing and Dr. Stephen S.Y. Lam for his proofreading. Thanks are extended to haematopathologists and clinical haematologists who have contributed to the diagnosis and management of patients described in this textbook. Some of the illustrations were generated using Servier Medical Art, provided by Servier and licensed under a Creative Commons Attribution 3.0 unported license.

Haemostasis and Thrombosis

1 Von Willebrand Disease

1.1 CLINICAL SCENARIO

A 7-year-old boy presented with easy bruising since infancy and had recurrent nose bleeding, requiring hospitalisations. His grandfather, father and one paternal aunt also had easy bruising. Physical examination was otherwise unremarkable.

1.2 LABORATORY REPORTS

	Results	References	Units
Platelet count	412	150–400	10^9/L
Prothrombin time	12.2	11.3–13.5	Seconds
Activated partial thromboplastin time (APTT)	37.1	25.9–33.7	Seconds
Factor VIII	0.36	0.5–1.5	I.U./mL
Von Willebrand Factor antigen	0.19	0.5–2.0	I.U./mL
Von Willebrand Factor ristocetin cofactor	0.01	0.5–1.5	I.U./mL

1.3 QUESTIONS

1. What is the likely diagnosis?
2. What further investigations are needed?
3. What is the management plan?

1.4 CLINICAL PROGRESS

A personal and family history of bleeding, a low level of Von Willebrand Factor (VWF) antigen and activity, and a lowish level of Factor (F) VIII supported the diagnosis of Von Willebrand Disease (VWD). A disproportionally low VWF activity with respect to VWF antigen suggested VWD Type 2. VWF multimer analysis by electrophoresis showed the absence of large molecular weight multimers (Figure 1.1A), suggesting Type 2A or B disease. Ristocetin-induced platelet aggregation (RIPA) test was negative with low dose ristocetin, excluding Type 2B disease. The diagnosis was VWD Type 2A.

A Desmopressin (DDAVP) test was performed.

	0 minute	60 minutes	120 minutes
Activated partial thromboplastin time (Seconds)	43.1	28.3	31.3
Factor VIII (IU/mL)	0.3	0.99	0.73
Von Willebrand Factor antigen (IU/mL)	0.14	0.46	0.38
Von Willebrand factor ristocetin cofactor (IU/mL)	0.01	0.14	0.09

DOI: 10.1201/9781003325413-2

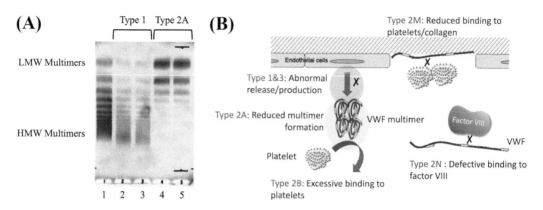

FIGURE 1.1 (A) Von Willebrand Factor (VWF) multimeric study. Lane 1: Normal control; Lanes 2, 3: A patient with Type 1 Von Willebrand Disease (VWD) showing reduced amounts of VWF multimers of all molecular weights; Lanes 4, 5: The index patient with Type 2A VWD showing a selective loss of high molecular weight multimers. LMW: Low molecular weight; HMW: High molecular weight. (B) Pathogenesis of VWD and its subtypes. (*Figure 1.1A, courtesy of Dr. Jason So.*)

When he had nose bleeding, subcutaneous DDAVP seemed to be effective in stopping bleeding. At the age of 17 years, he had a scheduled wisdom tooth extraction and was given plasma derived FVIII, VWF complex containing FVIII (250 IU) and VWF (500 IU) 1 hour before and 8 hours after the procedures. Intravenous transamin was also given prophylactically. The procedure was uneventful. At the age of 19 years, he developed right knee swelling after playing basketball. Magnetic resonance imaging showed haemarthrosis and ruptured anterior cruciate ligament and meniscus. He underwent surgery and was given FVIII and VWF complex and intravenous transamin, and the procedure was uneventful. He was largely asymptomatic thereafter.

1.5 VON WILLEBRAND FACTOR (VWF)

VWF is a large multimeric glycoprotein that is synthesised and released by vascular endothelial cells and activated platelets. It serves two physiological functions. It is essential for platelet adhesion to endothelial collagen during primary haemostasis. It also binds to and protects FVIII from degradation by activated protein C, thereby extending its half-life. Differential defects of these functions account for the clinical heterogeneity of VWD (Figure 1.1B).

1.6 VON WILLEBRAND DISEASE (VWD)

VWD is the most common inherited bleeding disorder, occurring in about 1 in 100 patients. It is a heterogeneous group of diseases with distinct molecular defects of VWF, laboratory features and clinical presentations, and they share in common abnormal haemostasis due to defective VWF functions. Unlike haemophilia, VWD is mostly inherited in an autosomal dominant manner, affecting male and female patients equally with females more likely to be symptomatic during menstruation and childbirth. Both quantitative (Types 1 & 3) and qualitative abnormalities (Type 2) are involved in VWF.

Type 1 VWD is the most common type (~ 75%) and results from a reduced release of VWF that is structurally normal. Mutations or deletion of the *VWF* gene can be identified in two-thirds of cases, and no detectable *VWF* gene mutation is identified in one-third of cases. It is autosomal-dominant with variable penetrance. A specific subtype known as Type 1C is characterised by a single nucleotide mutation, leading to increased clearance of VWF by macrophages. **Type 2 VWD** encompasses four distinct subtypes arising from qualitative defects of VWF and accounts for 20% of all VWD. **Type 2A** is the most common type and results from mutations that lead to reduced

VWF multimers. **Type 2B** results from gain-of-function mutation at a site that allows VWF multimers to interact with platelet glycoprotein 1b-alpha (GPIbα) spontaneously, leading to the rapid clearance of VWF multimers and platelets. **Type 2M** mutations span over a region in the *VWF* gene that encompasses loss-of-function mutation that impairs VWF binding not only to platelet GPIbα but also to collagen types I and III. Types 2A, 2B and 2M are inherited in an autosomal dominant fashion. **Type 2N** is caused by the abnormal binding of VWF to Factor VIII, leading to unstable and, hence a low level of FVIII. Unlike other subtypes, Type 2N is autosomal recessive and results from either a homozygous or compound heterozygous state. **Type 3 VWD** is a rare (5%) and severe disorder characterised by the complete absence of VWF. It is autosomal recessive, resulting from homozygous (or a compound heterozygote) null mutations.

1.7   DIAGNOSIS

The first clue to the diagnosis of VWD should be a personal or family history of bleeding tendency. Initial investigations including complete blood count, prothrombin time (PT) and activated partial thromboplastin time (APTT) serve as screening but are of little diagnostic value. Although prolonged APTT is typical of severe VWD, a normal APTT does not rule out VWD. Specific investigations include VWF antigen and surrogates of VWF functions including VWF ristocetin cofactor (VWF:RCo) and FVIII. A reduced VWF antigen (VWF:Ag) or VWF:Rco < 0.5 IU/mL should prompt the diagnosis of VWD. VWF:RCo/VWF:Ag ratio > 0.7 suggests Type 1, whereas that of < 0.7 suggests Type 2. Loss of high molecular weight multimers, as evaluated by gel electrophoresis, is indicative of Types 2A or 2B, whereas a normal pattern of multimers is consistent with Type 2M. A positive RIPA test in response to low dose ristocetin would support Type 2B. A relatively normal VWF:Ag and VWF:RCo and reduced FVIII should prompt the diagnosis of Type 2N. This type can be distinguished from haemophilia A by its autosomal inheritance. DDAVP challenge testing is indicated after the diagnosis of VWD has been established to evaluate if the treatment would be adequate for haemostasis. Response is adequate if there is a 2–4-fold increase in VWF:Ag and VWF:RCo and ≥ 30% sustained increase in FVIII levels. Adequate response is seen in 90% of patients with Type 1 VWD in whom DDAVP may suffice for the prophylactic management of bleeding associated with minor bleeding or procedures. Response is variable in Type 2 and absent in Type 3 VWD. The test is contraindicated in Type 2B VWD, as it may promote the binding of secreted VWF to platelets *in vivo* and worsen thrombocytopenia.

1.8   DIFFERENTIAL DIAGNOSIS

An important differential diagnosis of VWD is acquired Von Willebrand Syndrome, a secondary bleeding disorder with multiple mechanisms. In patients with aortic stenosis or other valvular disorders, the shearing of high molecular weight VWF multimers by mechanical stress or proteolysis may produce features reminiscent of Type 2A VWD. In patients with lymphoma, plasma cell dyscrasia or essential thrombocytosis, VWF may be absorbed by tumour cells and excessive platelets. In patients with autoimmune disease including systemic lupus erythematosus, autoantibody against VWF has been reported.

1.9   MANAGEMENT

Management of patients with VWD entails VWF replacement, stimulation of endogenous release and supportive care. Indication and schedule of VWF replacement depend on the severity and frequency of clinical bleeding. Patients with frequent and severe bleeding should receive prophylactic therapy, while those with occasional bleeding should receive on-demand therapy. Plasma-derived VWF is commonly used, and many preparations contain FVIII. Desmopressin, a synthetic version of vasopressin, stimulates the release of endogenous VWF and FVIII from endothelial cells. Typically, desmopressin increases VWF and FVIII levels to 2–4 times of baseline about 30–60 minutes after intravenous (IV) infusion or subcutaneous (SC) injection. It is ineffective in Type 3, which lacks endogenous VWF, Type 1C, in which a rise in VWF is characteristically short-lived or Types 2A or 2M, which produce dysfunctional VWF. Desmopressin is contraindicated in Type 2B, in which the release of defective VWF may increase binding to platelets and aggravate thrombocytopenia. Desmopressin trial can be considered for Types 1 and 1C. FVIII and VWF levels are commonly assessed at baseline and at 1 and 4 hours post-infusion. Response is defined by an increase of at least 2 times baseline VWF activity and sustained increase of FVIII and VWF above 0.50 IU/mL for at least 4 hours. Supportive treatments include the use of anti-fibrinolytic agent tranexamic acid and avoidance of contact sports and injuries.

1.10 KEY POINTS

1. VWD is the most common inherited bleeding disorder, resulting in quantitative (Types 1 and 3) and qualitative defects (Type 2) of VWF.
2. Haematological defects of VWD Type 2 depend on the sites of mutations. Those of Type 2N show remarkable similarity to haemophilia A but can be distinguished readily by a detailed family history.
3. VWD management entails VWF replacement, stimulation of endogenous release and supportive care. Exact treatment depends on the severity of bleeding and disease subtype.

ADDITIONAL READINGS

1. Weyand AC, Flood VH. Von Willebrand disease current status of diagnosis and management. Hematol Oncol Clin N Am 2021; 35: 1085–1101.
2. Harris NS, Pelletier JP, Marin MJ, Winter WE. Von Willebrand factor and disease: a review for laboratory professionals. Crit Rev Clin Lab Sci 2022; 59(4): 241–256.

2 Severe Haemophilia

2.1 CLINICAL SCENARIO

A 22-year-old man was referred to the haematology clinic for long-term follow up as his family immigrated to Hong Kong. He was born in Mainland China and presented with joint swelling when he was 6 months old. He has learnt to administer antihaemophilic globulin (AHG) by himself and has required 20–40 vials per month. He has developed recurrent right knee swelling and bilateral knee stiffness and a few episodes of gross haematuria. Gene sequencing showed inversion of the intron 22 of Factor (F) VIII. His younger brother has been having similar bleeding problems.

2.2 LABORATORY REPORTS

	Results	References	Units
Prothrombin time	14.4	11.3–13.2	Seconds
Activated partial thromboplastin time	71.5	27.6–37.6	Seconds
Platelet count	230	154–371	10^9/L
Factor VIII inhibitor	0	0	Bethesda unit
Hepatitis B surface antigen	Negative	Negative	
Anti-hepatitis C virus antibody	Negative	Negative	
Anti-human immunodeficiency virus antibody	Negative	Negative	

2.3 QUESTIONS

1. What is the diagnosis?
2. What is the management plan?
3. What are the long-term complications arising from this disease and its treatments?

2.4 HAEMOPHILIA A

Haemophilia A is an inherited bleeding disorder characterised by a deficiency of FVIII, which is encoded by the *F8* gene in the X-chromosome. It occurs in about 1 in 5,000 live male births. The clinical presentations are variable and depend on severity, which can be severe (FVIII activity < 1% or < 1 IU/dL), intermediate (1–5% or 1–5 IU/dL) or mild (> 5% or > 5 IU/dL). Severe cases usually present in the first 2 years of life with spontaneous musculoskeletal, soft tissue or life-threatening bleeding such as intracranial haemorrhage. Repeated intra-articular bleedings lead to severe, progressive, destructive and deformative arthropathy. Diagnosis is made in a male patient with bleeding tendency and low FVIII but normal Von Willebrand Factor (VWF) activities and can be confirmed by identification of the hemizygous *F8* pathogenic variant upon molecular genetic testing. The coagulation pathways are shown in Figure 2.1.

2.5 GENETICS

Haemophilia A is inherited as an X-linked recessive disorder. The majority of symptomatic patients are male who are hemizygous for the *F8* pathogenic variant. Females are heterozygous and are generally asymptomatic carriers, although some of them may have bleeding risk. For a male patient

DOI: 10.1201/9781003325413-3

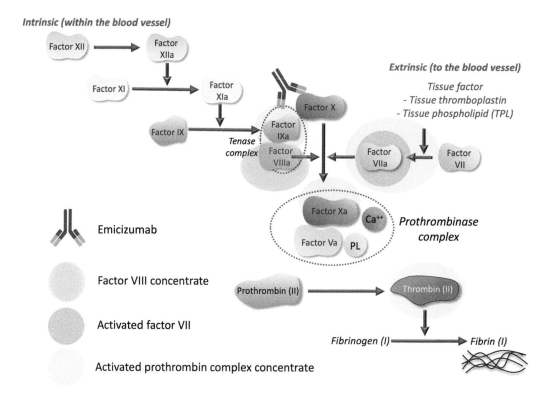

FIGURE 2.1   Coagulation pathways and the therapeutic options for severe haemophilia A. PL: Phospholipid.

planning to have children, he will transmit the *F8* pathogenic variant to all of his daughters, who will become carriers, and to none of his sons. For a female carrier, the chance of transmitting the *F8* pathogenic variant to her offspring will be 50%. The affected sons will be hemizygous and become haemophilic, whereas the affected daughters will be heterozygous carriers. Once the *F8* variant has been identified in the proband, genetic testing for at-risk family members, prenatal testing for a pregnancy at increased risk and preimplantation genetic testing are possible.

2.6   GENETIC TESTING

Genetic testing for patients with clinical and laboratory features of haemophilia A should be performed to confirm the diagnosis. The diverse genetic variations of *F8* necessitate a multi-pronged approach in the molecular diagnosis of haemophilia A. It entails polymerase chain reaction-based technologies targeting inversions involving **intron 22 or intron 1 of *F8***, which are detectable in nearly 50% of patients with severe haemophilia A but in none with moderate or mild cases. It should also be performed for potential female carriers with a family history of severe haemophilia A. In negative cases, gene-targeted next generation sequencing (NGS) should be performed to detect **small intragenic deletions or insertions and missense, nonsense and splice site variants.** Pathogenic variants can be detectable in 50% of severe cases and most of the mild and moderate cases. However, as **whole exon or whole-gene deletions or duplications** are typically missed with the NGS approach, gene-targeted deletion/duplication analysis based on multiplex ligation-dependent probe amplification (MLPA) should be performed for patients without identifiable genetic lesions.

2.7   DIFFERENTIAL DIAGNOSIS

A detailed personal and family history is needed to ascertain the inherited nature of this bleeding disorder. An important differential diagnosis is Von Willebrand Disease (VWD), which is the most common inherited bleeding disorder. In most circumstances, haemophilia A can be distinguished from VWD based on FVIII and Von Willebrand Factor (VWF) antigen and activity assays. An exception is VWD Type 2N, which shows normal VWF and a low FVIII level that makes it indistinguishable from mild haemophilia A. The latter can be ascertained by its X-linked recessive inheritance based on family history. These disorders can also be distinguished through molecular genetic testing or by measuring the binding of FVIII to VWF using enzyme-linked immunosorbent assay or column chromatography.

2.8   MANAGEMENT

General principle. Management of haemophilia entails collaboration among the medical, surgical and nursing teams in tertiary referral centres with expertise in inherited bleeding disorders. Replacement of FVIII is core to the management, which can be given on demand during bleeding episodes and prophylactically, particularly for patients with severe deficiency in whom bleeding is anticipated. Regular surveillance for alloimmune FVIII inhibitor is recommended, which occurs in 30% of patients receiving FVIII replacement. Patient education about precautions to avoid bleeding is important, and extended family screening of the proband should be performed.

FVIII concentrates. These are virally inactivated plasma-derived products made from plasma donated by human blood donors or recombinant products manufactured using genetically engineered cells and recombinant technology. They are comparable in efficacy. In the absence of FVIII inhibitor, each international unit (IU) of FVIII per kilogram of body weight infused intravenously will raise the plasma FVIII level by approximately 2 IU/dL. Therefore, the dosage of required Factor VIII equals the desired plasma level (IU/dL) x body weight (Kg) × 0.5. Peak plasma level is achieved 15–30 minutes after infusion. The half-life is approximately 12 hours; therefore, repeated dosing is needed for haemostasis during bleeding episodes or invasive surgery. Fusion (Fc-fusion; Albumin-fusion) and PEGylation forms are now available to extend the half-life of FVIII to reduce the frequency of administration. Fusion rescues endocytosed FVIII from intracellular degradation via interaction with the neonatal Fc receptor. PEGylation reduces FVIII interaction with the clearance of receptors.

Bypassing agents. Bypassing agents are used for the treatment and prevention of bleeding in patients with haemophilia A who develop anti-FVIII alloantibodies (inhibitors). Recombinant activated factor VIIa (rFVIIa) is a bypassing agent that binds to tissue factor to activate FX and FIX and allows the coagulation cascade to resume. Activated prothrombin complex concentrate (aPCC, aka FEIBA, Factor Eight Inhibitor Bypassing Activity) contains activated FII, FVII, FIX and FX.

Non-factor replacement therapy. Emicizumab is a chimeric bi-specific antibody directed against the enzyme FIXa and the zymogen FX and promotes FIXa-catalysed FX activation and tenase formation, mimicking the cofactor function of FVIII. Emicizumab is given subcutaneously and is characterised by its long half-life and high efficacy in the prevention of bleeding in patients with or without FVIII inhibitors. It is not intended to treat acute bleeding episodes.

Novel therapy under investigation. Haemostasis depends on the balance between procoagulants (e.g., clotting factors) and natural anticoagulants (e.g., antithrombin, tissue factor pathway inhibitor [TFPI] and activated protein C). Although haemophilia has been treated by replacing the missing procoagulant protein, inhibition of the natural anticoagulants is being explored as an alternative means to restore haemostasis. Fitusiran is an RNA interference therapy that specifically targets antithrombin mRNA to suppress the production of antithrombin in the liver. This therapy has the advantage of subcutaneous administration and prolonged duration of action, and due to its mechanism of action, it could be used in both haemophilia A and B patients with or without inhibitors. Anti-TFPI antibodies bind to the K2 domain or to both the K1 and K2 domains of TFPI, thus rescuing FXa and FVIIa from inhibition. These therapies can also be administered subcutaneously and restore haemostasis in both haemophilia A and B patients with or without inhibitors. Gene therapy for haemophilia based on viral transduction of Factor VIII is actively being tested in clinical trials. Haemophilia is ideally suitable for this treatment as a monogenic disease resulting from the deficiency of a single factor in which replacement of small amount of it can result in clinical improvement.

2.9 KEY POINTS

1. Haemophilia A results from genetic aberration of the *F8* gene in the X-chromosome, leading to FVIII deficiency.
2. Heterogeneous genetic aberrations in different patients result in variable severity of clinical manifestations.
3. Management of haemophilia A should be multi-disciplinary, and in addition to FVIII replacement, bypassing agents and bi-specific monoclonal antibodies are available. Novel therapeutic approaches are being evaluated.

ADDITIONAL READINGS

1. Konkle BA, Fletcher NS. Hemophilia A. In: Adam MP, Everman DB, Mirzaa GM et al., eds. *GeneReviews®*. University of Washington 1993–2022 [Internet]. 2000 Sep 21 [Updated 2022 Oct 27].
2. Nathwani AC. Gene therapy for hemophilia. Hematology Am Soc Hematol Educ Program 2022 Dec 9; 2022(1): 569–578.
3. Srivastava A, Santagostino E, Dougall A et al. WFH guidelines for the management of hemophilia. Haemophilia 2020 Aug; 26(Suppl 6): 1–158.

3 Factor VII Deficiency

3.1 CLINICAL SCENARIO

A 76-year-old woman had carcinoma of the cervix and laparoscopic total hysterectomy and bilateral salpingo-oophorectomy 10 years ago and appendicectomy 8 years ago. Both operations were uncomplicated. However, she recalled having an injection before surgery to prevent bleeding. She was married but had no children. She was referred to the haematology clinic for abnormal blood tests but was otherwise asymptomatic. Her younger sister died of uncontrolled bleeding after hysterectomy 30 years ago. Her elder sister was being followed up in the haematology clinic for a bleeding disorder.

3.2 LABORATORY REPORTS

	Results	Reference range	Units
Prothrombin time	56.4	10.9–13.6	Seconds
International normalised ratio	5.1	1	
Activated partial thromboplastin time	28.1	25.1–33.9	Seconds

3.3 QUESTIONS

1. What further investigation is needed?
2. What is the likely diagnosis?
3. What is the management plan?

3.4 PROGRESS

She had further investigations with respect to prolonged prothrombin time (PT).

	Results	Reference range	Units
Factor VII	0.02	0.5–1.5	IU/mL
Factor II	1.23	0.5–1.5	IU/mL
Factor V	1.23	0.5–1.5	IU/mL
Factor X	1.2	0.5–1.5	IU/mL

There was no evidence of immediate acting or time-dependent inhibitory activity detected by a PT-based inhibitor screen. A diagnosis of Factor (F) VII deficiency was made.

3.4.1 FACTOR VII (FVII)

FVII is a free-circulating glycoprotein of the serine protease family. It is one of the vitamin K-dependent proteins and is synthesised exclusively by the liver. Its half-life is extremely short (4–6 hours) and plasma level is 10 times less than other vitamin K-dependent factors. A small proportion (1%-3%) of circulating FVII exists as its activated form (FVIIa) in the absence of

DOI: 10.1201/9781003325413-4

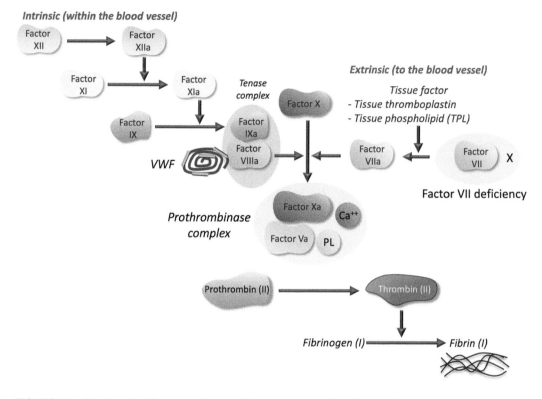

FIGURE 3.1 Physiological function of Factor VII in haemostasis. PL: Phospholipid; VWF: Von Willebrand Factor.

coagulation activation. Following injury, FVIIa binds to tissue factor (TF), and the FVIIa–TF complex generates a burst of activated FXa from FX, resulting in thrombin generation and formation of a fibrin clot (Figure 3.1).

3.4.2 FACTOR VII DEFICIENCY

Diagnosis of FVII deficiency is defined by an isolated prolonged PT and a low FVII level. FVII deficiency is autosomal recessive in inheritance. Two types of deficiency have been reported. Type I is quantitative, and Type II is qualitative due to mutations. To date, more than 250 mutations have been reported. Typically, a homozygous or compound heterozygous genotype is associated with a low FVII level < 10% (severe deficiency), whereas a heterozygous genotype is associated with a FVII level between 20 and 60%.

3.5 CLINICAL PRESENTATION

Clinical penetrance of inherited FVII deficiency is highly variable. There is no predictable and preferential site of bleeding, and bleeding risk does not correlate well with the level of deficiency or mutation sites. Intriguingly, venous thromboembolism (VTE) has been reported in patients with FVII deficiency. A causal relationship has not been ascertained, but the observations support at least the proposition that FVII deficiency does not protect patients from VTE.

3.6   TREATMENT

Patients with FVII deficiency who bleed should be treated with recombinant activated FVII concentrate. Given the lack of correlation between FVII and bleeding severity, routine monitoring of FVIIa activity is not warranted. If FVIIa is unavailable, then an alternative option is 4-factor prothrombin complex concentrate or fresh frozen plasma. This patient was given FVIIa prior to her previous surgeries.

3.7   DIFFERENTIAL DIAGNOSIS

An important differential diagnosis is coagulopathy involving different clotting factors. As FVII has the shortest half-life among all clotting factors, it is often the first to be depleted in conditions that affect multiple clotting factors, including liver failure, vitamin K deficiency and consumptive coagulopathy, *viz.*, disseminated intravascular coagulopathy. Acquired and isolated FVII deficiency is extremely rare, and when it happens, it is due to the presence of inhibitors secondary to malignancies. A detailed family and personal history is of the utmost importance to ascertain the hereditary nature of the disease.

3.8   KEY POINTS

1. Isolated prolongation of PT could be secondary to specific FVII deficiency or more commonly, multiple clotting factors deficiency due to liver failure, vitamin K deficiency or consumptive coagulopathy.
2. Clinical penetrance of inherited FVII deficiency is highly variable from being asymptomatic to having a high bleeding risk. Both quantitative and qualitative defects due to gene mutations have been described. There is no correlation with the FVII level or mutation sites.
3. In bleeding patients, FVIIa is the mainstay of treatment. An alternative option is 4-factor prothrombin complex concentrate or fresh frozen plasma.

ADDITIONAL READING

1. Sevenet PO, Kaczor DA, Depasse F. Factor VII deficiency: from basics to clinical laboratory diagnosis and patient management. Clin Appl Thromb/Hemost 2017; 23(7): 703–710.

4 Acquired Haemophilia

4.1 CLINICAL SCENARIO

An 82-year-old man presented with easy bruising in April 2021. He had pulmonary tuberculosis when he was 20 years old and carcinoma of the prostate 5 years ago, which was treated with radiotherapy. His previous blood results have been unremarkable.

4.2 LABORATORY REPORTS

	Results	Reference range	Units
Haemoglobin	12.7	13.3–17.1	g/dL
White cell count	7.10	3.89–9.93	10⁹/L
Platelet count	212	167–396	10⁹/L
Prothrombin time	11.8	10.9–13.6	Seconds
Activated partial thromboplastin time	90	25.1–33.9	Seconds

4.3 QUESTIONS

1. What is the next investigation?
2. What is the diagnosis?
3. What is the management approach?

4.4 CLINICAL PROGRESS

Further investigations included the following tests:

Lupus anticoagulant by dilute Russell's viper venom time (DRVVT) screen: Negative
Factors (F) IX, XI, XII levels: Normal
FVIII level < 0.01 IU/mL (Reference: 0.5–1.5 IU/mL)
FVIII inhibitor: 75.58 Bethesda unit (Reference: 0)
Inhibitor screening comment: Time-dependent inhibitory activity detected
Anti-nuclear factor: 1/160. Anti-double stranded DNA antibody and rheumatoid factor were negative.
Positron emission tomography/Computed tomography scan showed no fluorodeoxyglucose (FDG)-avid focus.

A diagnosis of acquired FVIII inhibitor was made. He was treated with oral tranexamic acid, cyclophosphamide, prednisolone and 4 weekly doses of rituximab in April 2021, resulting in normalisation of activated partial thromboplastin time (APTT) in two months (Figure 4.1A). FVIII inhibitor became undetectable three months after initial presentation.

4.5 ISOLATED APTT PROLONGATION

The interpretation of an isolated APTT prolongation is context-dependent. An important differential diagnosis is the presence of FXa inhibitor in patients receiving such treatments, for instance, low-molecular weight heparin and direct oral anticoagulant (DOAC), or patients whose blood samples

DOI: 10.1201/9781003325413-5

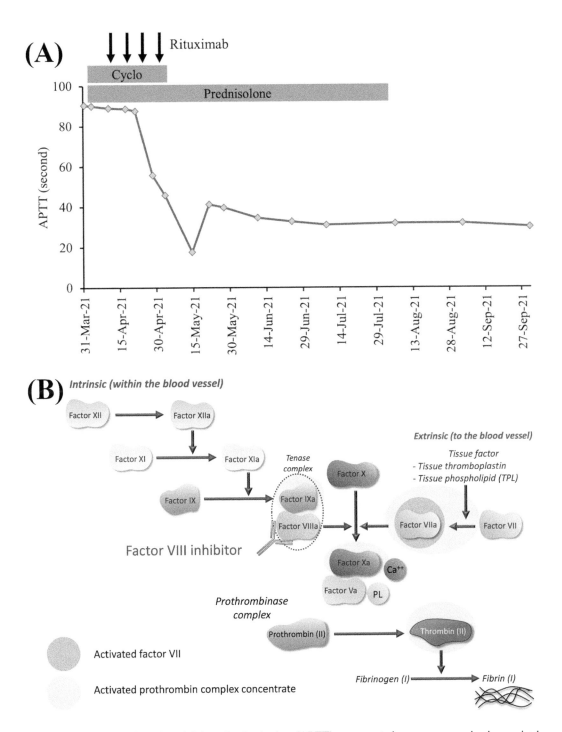

FIGURE 4.1 (A) Activated partial thromboplastin time (APTT) response to immunosuppression in acquired Factor (F) VIII inhibitor. Arrows indicate the rituximab doses. Cyclo: Cyclophosphamide. (B) Pathogenesis of acquired FVIII inhibitor and factor replacement options. Activated prothrombin complex concentrate comprises thrombin (FII), FVIIa, FIXa and FXa. Immunosuppressive therapy to reduce FVIII inhibitor is described in the text. PL: Phospholipid.

are contaminated by heparin. In the absence of drug treatment, isolated APTT prolongation in patients without bleeding tendency should raise the possibility of lupus anticoagulant. Another possibility is FXII deficiency, which in most cases, is identified incidentally but may occur in 2–3% of the general population. Both conditions may be associated with an increased risk of thrombosis rather than bleeding.

In a patient with a bleeding disorder, isolated APTT prolongation would suggest a defective intrinsic pathway, particularly FVIII and FIX. The new onset of bleeding and the previously normal blood results in this patient suggested an autoantibody (inhibitor) to the coagulation factors of the intrinsic pathway in which FVIII is most commonly affected. Bleeding that arises from acquired FVIII inhibitor can be severe. Unlike inherited FVIII deficiency, i.e., haemophilia A, which primarily affects joints, acquired FVIII inhibitor usually manifests as cutaneous, soft tissue, mucosal or muscle bleeding. Gastrointestinal and central nervous system (CNS) bleeding may also occur. In addition, although haemophilia A affects primarily boys and young males, acquired haemophilia shows no gender preponderance and affects mostly adult and elderly patients.

4.6   LABORATORY CONFIRMATION OF ACQUIRED FACTOR VIII INHIBITOR

Laboratory confirmation of acquired FVIII inhibitor requires both screening and definitive tests. A 1:1 mixing study is a widely used **screening test**. It is typically performed in two steps: Examination of immediate APTT correction and later at 1 and 2 hours at 37°C. In samples lacking FVIII, mixing with normal pooled plasma results in an immediate and complete correction of APTT. In samples carrying lupus anticoagulant, mixing cannot correct APTT despite prolonged incubation at 37°C due to the immediate and sustained inhibition of the intrinsic pathway. In contrast, acquired FVIII inhibitor is time- and temperature-dependent. Upon mixing with normal plasma, APTT is corrected immediately. However, later and at 37°C, the inhibitor becomes active, and APTT becomes prolonged again. **Definitive tests** of acquired FVIII inhibitor include a FVIII activity and inhibitor (Bethesda) assay. FVIII activity is reduced but detectable *in vitro* consistent with the second-order kinetics, but the residual activity *in vitro* is not clinically protective of bleeding. This contrasts with the allo-antibodies that occur in haemophilia A, which follow first-order kinetics. The Bethesda assay is used to determine the strength of the inhibitor, in which serial dilutions of patient plasma are incubated with normal pooled plasma for 2 hours at 37°C. FVIII activity is then measured at each dilution. The incubated control is considered to be 100% FVIII activity, and the reciprocal dilution of patient plasma that yields 50% FVIII activity is defined as a Bethesda unit (BU). For example, if the residual FVIII activity is 50% with a dilution of 1:10, then the actual inhibitor titre is 10 BU. Inhibitor titre ≥ 5 BU is generally considered high.

4.7   CAUSES OF ACQUIRED FACTOR VIII INHIBITOR

Acquired FVIII inhibitor is a rare disease, occurring in about 1 in a million people each year. Approximately 50% of cases of acquired FVIII inhibitor show no discernible cause. The remaining 50% happen mostly in the elderly or in the puerperal state. Cases occurring in the elderly are associated with malignancy, autoimmune disease or drug exposure including antibiotics, immunomodulatory drugs or anti-epileptics. The pathogenesis of acquired FVIII inhibitor generation is currently unclear.

4.8   TREATMENT

The rarity of the acquired FVIII inhibitor has precluded prospective evaluation and comparison of management strategies. Generally, treatment of bleeding diathesis requires both haemostasis and the suppression of autoantibodies formation. To achieve haemostasis, FVIII bypassing agents include recombinant activated FVII (FVIIa) or activated prothrombin complex concentrate (aPCC).

FVIIa catalyses the activation of FX to FXa on the surface of activated platelets, leading to the generation of thrombin. Activated PCC is a plasma-derived concentrate containing FII, FVII, FIX and FX in both activated and inactivated forms, which generate FXa and, thus, thrombin (Figure 4.1B). Judicious use of these agents is needed as both can induce thrombosis inadvertently. Suppression of autoantibodies formation is usually achieved by corticosteroid, and response can be enhanced by the concomitant use of cyclophosphamide. More recently, rituximab, given as 4 weekly doses, is increasingly used as an adjunct to corticosteroid and cyclophosphamide and may give rise to a more sustained suppression of the inhibitor.

4.9   KEY POINTS

1. Isolated prolongation of APTT in a **bleeding** patient not taking FXa inhibitor suggests defective FVIII or FIX.
2. Diagnosis of acquired inhibitor to FVIII entails a 1:1 mixing study as a **screening test** and a FVIII activity and inhibitor (Bethesda) assay as **definitive tests.**
3. Treatment of acquired FVIII inhibitor requires both haemostasis and suppression of auto-antibodies formation.

ADDITIONAL READING

1. Pai M. Acquired hemophilia A. Hematol Oncol Clin N Am 2021; 35: 1131–1142.

5 Acquired Factor V Inhibitor

5.1 CLINICAL SCENARIO

An 81-year-old man with a history of hypertension and hypertensive nephropathy was admitted for community-acquired pneumonia, which was complicated by atrial fibrillation and pulmonary oedema. He received amoxicillin/clavulanic acid, azithromycin and amiodarone with clinical improvement. His prothrombin (PT) and activated partial thromboplastin time (APTT) were prolonged 2 weeks after admission. They were normal at presentation.

5.2 LABORATORY REPORTS

	Results	References	Units
Prothrombin time	34.7	11.3–13.2	Seconds
Activated partial thromboplastin time	42.9	27.6–37.6	Seconds
Thrombin time	20.7	20.9–23.9	Seconds
Fibrinogen	4.53	1.71–3.38	g/L

Liver function and complete blood count: Normal.

He was given daily intravenous vitamin K1 10 mg and fresh frozen plasma (FFP) with no response. There was no significant bleeding tendency. Antibiotics and amiodarone were stopped.

5.3 QUESTIONS

1. What are the next investigations?
2. What are the possible diagnoses?
3. What is the management plan?

5.4 CLINICAL PROGRESS

Initial investigations reported an isolated Factor (F) V deficiency of 0.12 IU/mL (Ref: 0.5–1.5 IU/mL). FII, FVII and FX levels were normal. An inhibitor screen by a 1:1 mixing study was negative. Lupus anticoagulant (LA) was present, but anti-cardiolipin and anti-ß2 glycoprotein I antibodies were negative. After an initial improvement for 3 weeks, his PT and APTT were further prolonged to 65.7 and 92.6 seconds, respectively. There was no significant bleeding except minor bruises over the venipuncture site. Laboratory investigations were repeated. FII, FVII and FX levels were normal, and FV remained deficient. A FV assay demonstrated non-parallelism between the patient's and the standard curves, which suggested an inhibitor. LA was again present. A repeat mixing study demonstrated an immediate acting inhibitor detectable by both the PT and APTT systems. The inhibitor titre was 5.8 Bethesda units. He was treated with prednisolone 1 mg/kg, and 4 weeks after treatment, his PT and APTT were normalised.

5.5 INTERPRETATION OF PROLONGED PT AND APTT

Prolonged PT and APTT could be secondary to multiple clotting factor deficiency. This is frequently seen in liver diseases, vitamin K deficiency or consumptive coagulopathy. More rarely, it could

DOI: 10.1201/9781003325413-6

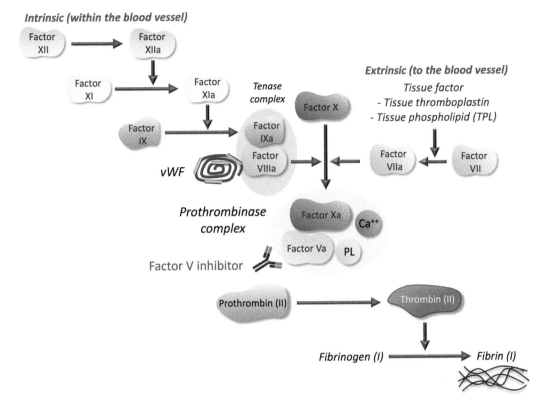

FIGURE 5.1 The coagulation pathway. Factor (F) Va forms an integral part of prothrombinase complex that catalyses the conversion of prothrombin to thrombin, leading to the formation of fibrin. Inhibitor to FVa perturbs the prothrombinase complex, leading to prolonged prothrombin time and activated partial thromboplastin time. PL: Phospholipid; VWF: Von Willebrand Factor.

be due to a deficiency of a single factor that is involved in the common coagulation pathway (Figure 5.1).

5.5.1 ACQUIRED FACTOR V INHIBITOR

5.5.1.1 Clinical Presentation and Association

Acquired FV inhibitor is rare, but it affects patients of all ages. Clinical symptoms are diverse, ranging from prolonged PT and APPT in asymptomatic patients to life-threatening bleeding. A notable risk factor is the exposure to bovine thrombin that is frequently used as topical haemostatic agents in vascular, orthopaedic and neurosurgical procedures. These agents often contain bovine proteins including FV that induce anti-bovine FV inhibitors, which cross-react with human FV. The risk has become lower due to the increasing use of recombinant thrombin for these purposes. Other risk factors include antibiotic exposure (especially of the β-lactam group), blood transfusions, cancers and autoimmune disorders.

5.5.1.2 Laboratory Abnormalities

Characteristically, both PT and APPT are prolonged. They are not correctible upon 1:1 mixing with normal plasma. Repeated testing may be necessary, as in this case. Unlike FVIII inhibitors, FV inhibitors act immediately in mixing studies and show no time dependence. Thrombin time (TT) is usually normal, except in the cases of FV inhibitors associated with prior bovine thrombin exposure (see previously) due to the presence of antibodies against bovine thrombin. Lupus anticoagulant may be present due to the interference of FV binding to the phospholipid membrane.

5.5.1.3 Management

Potential agents associated with FV inhibitor should be discontinued. Asymptomatic patients with FV inhibitor should be monitored closely and may not need treatment, as spontaneous resolution occurs in up to 40% of patients. Management of patients with bleeding complications entails haemostasis and suppression of inhibitor production. Platelet transfusion is the first line of treatment; this is predicated on the premise that a high concentration of FV may be released from α granules of platelets at the site of injury, and it has a greater procoagulant potential than plasma FV. It is also less susceptible to neutralisation by the FV inhibitor. Patients who do not respond well to platelet transfusion should receive additional therapy including activated prothrombin complex concentrate (aPCC) or activated recombinant FVII (rFVIIa). FXa derived from aPCC or generated by rFVIIa may bind to FV from platelets to achieve haemostasis. Production of FV inhibitor can be suppressed using immunosuppressive therapy including corticosteroid, cyclophosphamide or anti-CD20 antibody rituximab.

5.6   KEY POINTS

1. Prolonged PT and APTT could be secondary to multiple clotting factors deficiency, which occurs in liver diseases, vitamin K deficiency or consumptive coagulopathy. More rarely, it could be due to the deficiency of a single factor that is involved in the common coagulation pathway.
2. The presence of acquired FV inhibitor can be demonstrated by FV deficiency and an immediately acting inhibitor in a 1:1 mixing study.
3. Management of acquired FV inhibitor associated with bleeding complications includes cessation of the triggering agent, platelet transfusion and immunosuppression.

ADDITIONAL READING

1. Hirai D, Yamashita Y, Masunaga N et al. Acquired factor V inhibitor. Intern Med 2016; 55(20): 3039–3042.

6 Disseminated Intravascular Coagulopathy

6.1 CLINICAL SCENARIO

A 79-year-old man with hypertension, a hepatitis B carrier state and sick sinus syndrome was diagnosed as chronic type A aortic dissection since 2013. Repeated computed tomography scans showed a chronic dissection flap at the distal ascending aorta, and he was managed conservatively. He has been repeatedly admitted since 2015 for recurrent and unprovoked limb haematoma.

6.2 LABORATORY REPORTS

	Results	References	Units
Haemoglobin	11.1	13.3–17.1	g/dL
White cell count	5.7	3.89–9.93	10^9/L
Platelet count	68	154–371	10^9/L
Prothrombin time	15.9	10.6–13.6	Seconds
Activated partial thromboplastin time	30.7	25.1–33.9	Seconds
Fibrinogen	0.5	1.71–3.38	g/L
D-dimer	4.27	< 0.8	mg/L FEU*
Thrombin time	26.9	20.9–23.9	Seconds
Lactate dehydrogenase	232	118–221	IU/L

* Fibrinogen Equivalent Unit.
Blood film: Mild schistocytes and polychromasia. No dysplasia. Normal differential count.

6.3 QUESTIONS

1. What is the haematological abnormality?
2. What could be the underlying cause?
3. What is the management approach?

6.4 DIAGNOSIS

In this patient, the presence of thoracic aortic dissection, thrombocytopenia, a prolonged prothrombin time, reduced fibrinogen and raised D-dimer collectively supported the diagnosis of disseminated intravascular coagulopathy (DIC). DIC is not a disease but a manifestation of underlying, often severe, clinical conditions that lead to the activation of coagulation. These conditions include, among others, severe **infection**, particularly bacteraemia, advanced **malignancies**, for instance, metastatic adenocarcinoma and acute promyelocytic leukaemia, severe **trauma**, head injury or burns, **obstetric complications**, particularly abruptio placentae and amniotic fluid embolism, and **vascular abnormalities**, notably giant haemangioma and a large aortic aneurysm.

Thrombocytopenia is a consistent feature in DIC. Severe microangiopathic haemolytic anaemia should raise the suspicion of thrombotic thrombocytopenic purpura (TTP), although mild red cell fragmentation can also be seen in DIC. Evidence of consumptive coagulopathy, particularly of

DOI: 10.1201/9781003325413-7

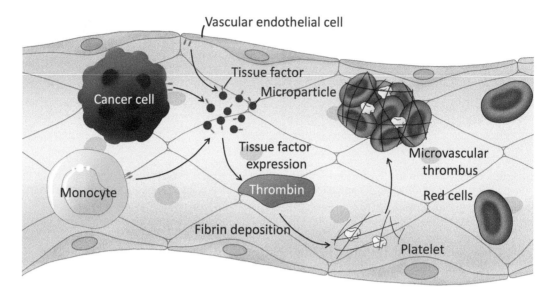

FIGURE 6.1 Pathogenesis of disseminated intravascular coagulopathy. The release of tissue factor from activated monocytes, vascular endothelial cells or cancer cells and the subsequent activation of the coagulation pathway are central to the pathogenesis.

prolonged PT and hypofibrinogenaemia, is characteristic of DIC. However, fibrinogen is an acute phase reactant, and a normal or raised fibrinogen level does not rule out DIC. Fibrin markers including D-dimer and fibrin degradation product are usually raised in DIC. None of these laboratory markers is diagnostic, and they must be interpreted in the relevant clinical context associated with DIC.

6.5 PATHOGENESIS

DIC arises from the abnormal initiation and propagation of the coagulation pathway. It begins with the **release of tissue factor** from activated monocytes, vascular endothelial cells or cancer cells (Figure 6.1). In aortic dissection, tissue factor is released from endothelial cells that are damaged by the turbulent blood flow, which activates the coagulation pathway. This results in thrombin generation and the subsequent fibrinogen to fibrin conversion, leading to microvascular thrombus formation. During this process, platelets become activated, and they release P-selectin, which further increases tissue factor expression from monocytes. The end result is the widespread activation of coagulation; this leads to the consumption of platelets and coagulation factors. As **thrombosis** ensues, organ perfusion may be compromised, leading to organ dysfunction. However, thrombocytopenia, reduced levels of clotting factors and high levels of fibrin degradation products may affect platelet function and fibrin cross-linking, which leads to **bleeding diathesis**. In addition, DIC is associated with **changes in the fibrinolytic pathways,** which are context-dependent. For instance, vascular abnormalities and acute promyelocytic leukaemia are characteristically associated with enhanced fibrinolysis due to increased tissue plasminogen activator (t-PA) and the conversion of plasminogen to plasmin, which is fibrinolytic. These patients are susceptible to bleeding rather than thrombosis. However, sepsis-related DIC is associated with an increase in plasminogen activator inhibitor-1 (PAI-1), which inhibits t-PA and suppresses fibrinolysis. These patients are susceptible to thrombosis.

6.6 MANAGEMENT OF DIC

In principle, DIC management should focus on the eradication of the underlying cause. Specific management of DIC depends on the clinical context, and in general, the goal is to prevent either thrombosis or bleeding arising from DIC. Patients at risk of thrombosis should receive anticoagulation in the absence of contraindications. However, patients with DIC who are at a high risk of bleeding should maintain haemostatic factors including the transfusion of platelets and fibrinogen concentrate. Fibrinolytic inhibitor, notably tranexamic acid, can also be used to treat or prevent bleeding.

6.7 KEY POINTS

1. Clinically, DIC is characterised by consumptive coagulopathy, leading to thrombocytopenia, prolonged prothrombin time/activated partial thromboplastin time and reduced fibrinogen.
2. The release of tissue factor from activated monocytes, vascular endothelial cells or cancer cells and the subsequent activation of the coagulation pathway is central to the pathogenesis of DIC.
3. Depending on the clinical context, patients with DIC may be at risk of thrombosis or bleeding.

ADDITIONAL READINGS

1. Levi M, Scully M. How I treat disseminated intravascular coagulopathy. Blood 2018; 131(8): 845–854.
2. Yamada S, Asakura H. Therapeutic strategies for disseminated intravascular coagulation associated with aortic aneurysm. Int J Mol Sci 2022; 23: 1296.

7 Cancer-Related Thrombosis

7.1 CLINICAL SCENARIO

A 72-year-old woman with a history of colonic polyps and diverticulosis presented with epigastric pain for three months. An upper endoscopy at a private clinic showed mild gastritis. Physical examination showed sinus tachycardia, mild tachypnoea at rest and mild fever at 38°C. There was mild epigastric tenderness.

7.2 LABORATORY REPORTS

	Results	References	Units
pH	7.52	7.35–7.45	
pO_2	9.2	10.4–14.0	kPa
pCO_2	3.9	4.7–6.0	kPa
Serum $pHCO_3^-$	24	22–26	mmol/L
Prothrombin time	18.2	11.3–13.2	Seconds
Activated partial thromboplastin time	29.1	27.6–37.6	Seconds
D-dimer	> 35.2	< 0.5	mg/L FEU*

* Fibrinogen Equivalent Unit

Her complete blood count and renal and liver function tests, except for a low serum albumin of 25 g/L (Reference: 39–50 g/L) and an elevated alkaline phosphatase of 346 U/L (reference: 47–124 U/L), were within normal limits.

7.3 QUESTIONS

1. What is the possible clinical condition?
2. What are the next investigations?
3. What is the management plan?

7.4 CLINICAL PROGRESS

Computed tomography (CT) of the abdomen showed a 3.9 × 4.3 × 4.6 cm irregular hypodense lesion at the pancreatic tail and multiple hypodense lesions in the liver. CT pulmonary angiogram showed multiple filling defects in both main pulmonary arteries (Figure 7.1). A diagnosis of pulmonary embolism (PE) with radiological evidence of carcinoma of the pancreatic tail was made. Serum CA19–9 was 691 U/mL (reference: < 37 U/mL). She received enoxaparin immediately, followed by apixaban. Her tachycardia, tachypnoea and fever subsided in a few days. She was referred to oncologists for the treatment of her underlying carcinoma of the pancreas.

7.5 PATHOGENESIS

Venous thromboembolism (VTE) encompasses a group of diseases including PE and deep vein thrombosis (DVT). DVT most often affects the lower limbs but can also occur in the upper limbs,

DOI: 10.1201/9781003325413-8

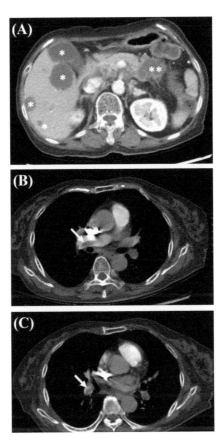

FIGURE 7.1 (A) Tumour masses in the tail of the pancreas (double asterisks) and in the liver (asterisk). (B) Filling defects in the pulmonary arterial trunk (arrow) and (C) segmental arteries (arrow).

cerebral and abdominal veins. Traditionally, the pathogenesis was explained based on the Virchow's triad, *viz.*, stasis, vessel wall damage and hypercoagulability. It is becoming clear that in VTE, the activation of endothelial cells induces the expression of selectins and Von Willebrand Factor, which bind circulating leukocytes and platelets (Figure 7.2). Activated leukocytes release microparticles that contain the procoagulant tissue factor, which activates Factor VII and initiates the extrinsic pathway. This is distinct from normal haemostasis in which tissue factor is released from subendothelial tissues upon injury. In addition, circulating neutrophils produce neutrophil extracellular traps (NETs), which contain DNA, histone and antimicrobial proteins, and generate a scaffold for red cells, platelets and procoagulant molecules to induce thrombosis. Extracellular DNA in NETs may also activate Factor XII and, thus, the intrinsic coagulation pathway. In cancer-associated thrombosis, cancer cells may express and release i) tissue factor and other procoagulant factors that activate the coagulation cascade; ii) inflammatory cytokines and carcinoma mucins that cause leukocyte and endothelial dysfunction; and iii) plasminogen activator inhibitor-1 that inhibits the natural fibrinolytic system.

7.6 RISK FACTORS OF VTE

The risk factors of VTE are diverse, and multiple factors may occur in a single VTE patient, suggesting that in these circumstances, VTE may be multi-factorial (Table 7.1). Importantly, active cancer at different stages of diseases accounts for 20% of VTE, and patients with active cancers

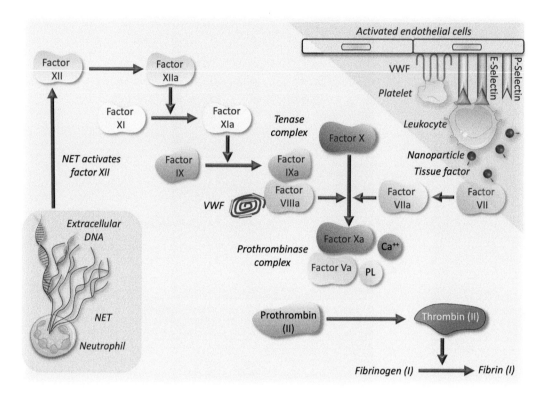

FIGURE 7.2 Pathogenesis of venous thromboembolism (VTE). Both the activation of Factor VII (right side) by tissue factor released from leukocytes and Factor XII by extracellular DNA in neutrophil extracellular traps (NETs) (left) contribute to the initiation of thrombosis. PL: Phospholipid; VWF: Von Willebrand Factor.

TABLE 7.1

Causes of Venous Thromboembolism

Hypercoagulability

Antiphospholipid syndrome

Blood diseases, e.g., paroxysmal nocturnal haemoglobinuria

Cancers

Drugs, e.g., L-asparaginase, thalidomide, heparin

OEstrogen, e.g., replacement, oral contraceptive pills

Familial, e.g., Factor V Leiden, prothrombin gene mutation, protein C, protein S and antithrombin deficiency

Pregnancy (Gravidity)

Haemolytic state

Iron deficiency anaemia

*JAK*2V617 positive myeloproliferative neoplasm

Stasis

Immobilisation

Compression, e.g., tumours, pregnancy

Vessel wall injury

Foreign device, e.g., central venous catheter

Post-trauma and surgery

have a 10 times higher risk of VTE than non-cancer patients, depending on the histological cancer types, specific oncogenic mutations, clinical stage of the disease and patient-related risk factors. Cancers arising from the gastrointestinal tract, particularly those of the pancreas and stomach, and cancers arising from the genitourinary tract, particularly those of the ovary and bladder, are associated with the highest prevalence of VTE. Among cancer patients, VTE is one of the leading causes of death, second after death related to cancer progression. Hereditary causes of VTE, notably Factor V Leiden and prothrombin gene mutations, are relatively rare in Chinese patients.

7.7 DIAGNOSIS OF VTE

The diagnosis of VTE was based on a high index of clinical suspicion and laboratory and radiological investigations. **Clinically**, patients with lower limb DVT characteristically present with swelling, pain and redness of the affected limb. Patients with PE present with shortness of breath, pleuritic chest pain or haemoptysis. Sinus tachycardia is usually present, and in severe case, patients may present with shock, syncope or sudden death. In all cases of VTE, fever is a common occurrence. About half of the patients with PE are associated with coexisting lower limb DVT. Clinical probability assessment tools are available to ascertain the likelihood of VTE based on clinical grounds. VTE may also occur at rare sites. Patients with VTE of the cerebral veins may present with headache, impaired consciousness, seizures or focal neurological signs. Abdominal vein thrombosis, including that of the hepatic, portal and mesenteric veins, may present with abdominal pain, ascites or impaired liver function and gastrointestinal tract bleeding. When it happens in previously unprovoked conditions, rare underlying causes should be screened for, e.g., paroxysmal nocturnal haemoglobinuria or polycythaemia vera. **In the laboratory**, D-dimer can be used to rule out VTE. D-dimer is the degradation product of cross-linked fibrin, and its level is increased during acute thrombosis. Although increased D-dimer can occur in various other conditions including cancer, infection, inflammation and pregnancy and is thus not diagnostic of VTE, a normal D-dimer level can help exclude significant VTE, particularly where the likelihood of VTE is low based on clinical grounds. **Radiological diagnosis** of VTE is essential, particularly in patients with a high clinical likelihood of VTE or those with positive D-dimer. For limb DVT, compression ultrasonography is the first line of radiological investigation, and for suspected PE, pulmonary CT angiography and ventilation-perfusion scintigraphy are gold standards for diagnosis, although the latter is becoming less popular in many centres.

7.8 TREATMENT

Traditionally, treatment of VTE entails low molecular weight heparin (LMWH) followed by warfarin, which is a vitamin K antagonist. Direct oral anticoagulants (DOACs), which include direct thrombin inhibitor (e.g., dabigatran) or Factor Xa inhibitor (e.g., rivaroxaban, edoxaban and apixaban), have revamped the treatment paradigm of VTE; generally, they are considered at least as effective as the conventional LMWH and warfarin regimen in preventing recurrent VTE and are generally associated with fewer major bleeding complications. However, the choice of treatment should be individualised with reference to the underlying clinical conditions and patient-specific factors.

In cancer-associated thrombosis, the continuation of LMWH has been shown to be more effective than warfarin in preventing VTE recurrence. Meta-analyses comparing LMWH with Factor Xa inhibitors showed that the latter were associated with a lower risk of VTE recurrence but a higher risk of major bleeding. Therefore, in cancer patients with a recent bleeding event or those who are at high risk of bleeding, LMWH may be preferred. Among the Factor Xa inhibitors, edoxaban and rivaroxaban are associated with a higher risk of bleeding in patients with gastrointestinal cancer, and in this circumstance, apixaban may be preferred. In patients with antiphospholipid syndrome, particularly those who are triple positive for lupus anticoagulant, anticardiolipin and anti-β2 glycoprotein I antibodies or those with very high antibody titres, VTE should be treated with LMWH and warfarin rather than DOACs as DOACs may be associated with a high risk of arterial thrombosis in clinical trials. In pregnancy-associated thrombosis, both warfarin and DOACs can cross placenta and are associated with adverse outcomes. Therefore, only LMWH can be used. During breast feeding, either warfarin and LMWH can be given, and DOACs should be avoided due to the lack of mature safety data in this setting. A number of patient factors should also be considered in the choice of anticoagulant. In patients with renal impairment with creatinine clearance of less than 30 mL/min, DOACs should be avoided due to their renal excretion. The safety and efficacy profiles of DOACs in obese patients are also less well-defined.

7.9   DURATION OF TREATMENT

In general, anticoagulation for VTE should be given for 3–6 months to reduce the risk of early recurrence. The decision on treatment continuation beyond 3–6 months is a risk-benefit consideration that balances the risk of VTE recurrence and major bleeding. Patients with ongoing VTE risk factors, e.g., active cancers, antiphospholipid syndrome and life-threatening VTE at presentation, and those who are not at a particularly high risk of major bleeding should be given long-term anticoagulation. Patients whose VTE risk factors have resolved, e.g., recovery from trauma or surgical operation or the cessation of oestrogen replacement or those who are at risk of major bleeding, should terminate anticoagulation after 3–6 months.

7.10   COMPLICATIONS OF VTE

Complications of VTE include the recurrence of thrombosis, bleeding during anticoagulation and post-thrombotic and post-PE syndrome. In particular, post-thrombotic syndrome, which occurs in up to one-third of patients with DVT, entails a spectrum of clinical manifestations due to chronic venous insufficiency that ranges from ankle swelling, venous claudication or leg ulcers. Post-PE syndrome can result in chronic thromboembolic pulmonary hypertension, which occurs in up to 3% of patients with PE.

7.11   KEY POINTS

1. Overall, 20% of VTE cases are associated with active cancers and are the second most common cause of death in these patients.
2. Diagnosis of VTE is based on clinical, laboratory and radiological features.
3. The choice of LMWH, warfarin and DOACs in VTE depends on the clinical context and the relative risk of bleeding and VTE recurrence.

ADDITIONAL READING

1. Khan F, Tritschler T, Kahn SR, Rodger MA. Venous thromboembolism. Lancet 2021; 398: 64–77.

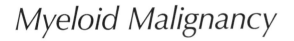

Myeloid Malignancy

8 Acute Myeloid Leukaemia I

8.1 CLINICAL SCENARIO

A 55-year-old man with good past health presented with shortness of breath and easy bruising for 1 week. He was married and has three children. He is the youngest of 3 siblings. There was no family history of blood diseases or malignancies. Except for pallor, physical examination was unremarkable.

8.2 LABORATORY REPORTS

	Results	References	Units
Haemoglobin	7.1	13.3–17.1	g/dL
White cell count	35	3.89–9.92	10^9/L
Platelet count	15	154–371	10^9/L

Blood smear showed circulating blasts of 5×10^9/L and promonocytes of 0.59×10^9/L. Bone marrow (BM) aspirate showed 30% blasts where Auer rods were readily identified (Figure 8.1A). The blasts were positive for myeloperoxidase and Sudan Black B staining. Cytogenetics showed t(8;21) translocation.

8.3 QUESTIONS

1. What is the diagnosis?
2. What is the management plan?
3. What is the prognosis?

8.4 CLINICAL PROGRESS

A diagnosis of acute myeloid leukaemia (AML) with t(8;21) translocation was made. The patient received induction chemotherapy comprising 7 days of cytarabine and 3 days of daunorubicin ("7+3" regimen) and achieved morphological remission. The chemotherapy was complicated by hepatosplenic microabscesses (Figure 8.1B), which resolved upon antifungal treatment. Thereafter, 4 courses of high-dose cytarabine consolidation was given. Minimal (measurable) residual disease (MRD) monitoring was performed based on detection of *RUNX1::RUNX1T1* fusion caused by t(8;21) translocation using quantitative reverse transcription polymerase chain reaction (Figure 8.1C). There was a period of negative MRD after chemotherapy, and the patient was closely monitored. Shortly thereafter, there was a resurgence of *RUNX1::RUNX1T1* transcript, and the patient was referred for allogeneic haematopoietic stem cell transplantation (HSCT) from his haploidentical daughter. The transplantation was complicated by cytokine release syndrome, which was treated by tocilizumab, a monoclonal antibody against interleukin-6 receptor. He subsequently developed graft-versus-host disease (GVHD) of the skin, liver and gut, requiring intensification of immunosuppression, including systemic corticosteroid. His MRD has remained negative since then.

DOI: 10.1201/9781003325413-10

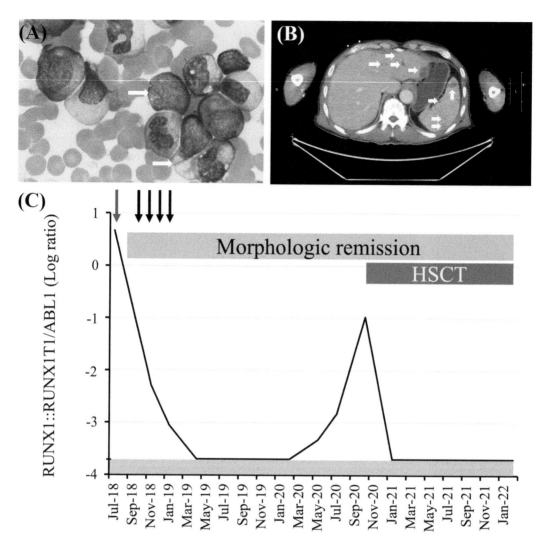

FIGURE 8.1 (A) Bone marrow aspirate showing an increased number of blasts and the presence of slender Auer rods inside their cytoplasm (arrows). There was evidence of granulocytic maturation (Wright-Giemsa × 1000). (B) Development of hepatosplenic microabscesses (arrows) due to candidiasis resulting from prolonged neutropenia. (C) Minimal (measurable) residual disease (MRD) based on detection of *RUNX1::RUNX1T1* fusion transcript. Red arrow: Induction chemotherapy; Black arrows: Consolidation chemotherapy. There was a resurgence of MRD, which is a harbinger of frank haematological relapse. MRD was rendered negative after allogeneic haematopoietic stem cell transplantation (HSCT).

8.5   ACUTE MYELOID LEUKAEMIA—DIAGNOSIS

AML is a disease of diverse clinicopathologic, cytogenetic and genetic characteristics, but it shares in common an abnormal increase in circulating or BM blasts of myeloid lineage. **Morphologically**, the blasts are characterised by a high nucleus-to-cytoplasm ratio, prominent nucleoli and open chromatic texture. A cut-off of 20% blasts in blood or BM is a general prerequisite to the diagnosis of AML. Characteristically, Auer rods are present in the cytoplasm, arising from abnormal fusion of azurophilic granules. These structures are pathognomonic of AML and are absent in blasts of lymphoblastic leukaemia or those arising from reactive BM changes. Typically, the blasts are positive for **cytochemical staining**, including myeloperoxidase and Sudan Black B staining. In cases where myeloid lineage specification of the blasts is not apparent, **immunophenotyping** by flow cytometry is needed. Once a diagnosis is made, **cytogenetics** by conventional karyotyping and **genetic analysis** by gene specific PCR or next generation sequencing (NGS) of a panel of mutations recurrent in myeloid malignancies are essential for prognostication. Some of the cytogenetic and genetic abnormalities, including but not limited to t(8;21) translocation, inv(16) and *NPM1* mutations, are considered pathognomonic of AML, and the 20% diagnostic prerequisite is lifted for these cases.

8.6 CLINICAL PRESENTATION

The incidence of AML increases with age, with a median age of onset at about 65 years. Typically, patients present with symptoms associated with BM failure, including anaemia, bleeding and infection. Rarely, patients may present with extramedullary diseases, known as myeloid sarcoma. Some patients may have an antecedent history of myelodysplastic syndrome (MDS) or myeloproliferative neoplasm (MPN), and AML could result from leukaemic transformation of these diseases (secondary AML). AML in patients with prior exposure to genotoxic agents are known as therapy-related AML (t-AML), and those with a family history of myeloid diseases and proven germline transmission of specific gene mutation are defined as myeloid malignancies with germline predisposition. AML in patients without such personal or family history are known as *de novo* AML.

8.7 PROGNOSTICATION

The diverse clinicopathologic, cytogenetic and genetic features of AML and the one-size-fits-all approach based on induction and consolidation chemotherapy result in different treatment outcomes. According to patients' diagnostic cytogenetic and genetic characteristics, the disease can be divided into favourable, intermediate or adverse risk groups, which reflects their differential sensitivity to chemotherapy. Prognostication is important for patient counselling at diagnosis and for guiding a decision on HSCT upon first complete remission (CR).

8.8 MRD MONITORING

For a typical patient with AML, there may be up to 10^{12} leukaemia cells in the body at diagnosis. Although morphologic complete remission (CR) is a prerequisite for long-term survival, the leukaemia load is estimated to be 10^9 at CR after induction chemotherapy, representing a substantial residual disease that may become the basis of future relapse. MRD detection is predicated on the premise that by using detection platforms with substantially higher sensitivity, the depth of response can be evaluated in real time, and the information can be used to inform prognosis and guide decision on HSCT at morphologic CR. At present, MRD can be assessed based on flow cytometry and molecular means. A persistently negative MRD is considered evidence of disease eradication.

8.9 MANAGEMENT OF AML

The management of AML focuses on disease eradication and the prevention of complications, and complications are the major cause of morbidity and mortality in patients. Young and fit patients are treated with "7+3" induction, which comprises 7 days of cytarabine and 3 days of anthracycline, typically daunorubicin. On average, 70–80% of patients achieve morphologic remission. These patients should receive high-dose cytarabine as consolidation. The contention is often the decision on HSCT at the first CR. In general, patients with favourable cytogenetic and genetic features at diagnosis may be closely monitored without HSCT to avoid HSCT toxicity. Patients with intermediate and adverse features should be considered for allogeneic HSCT to prevent relapse, if donors are available. A persistently positive MRD or a rising MRD post-chemotherapy is considered a harbinger of frank haematological relapse, and such patients should receive allogeneic HSCT. Old and unfit patients who are not candidates for intensive chemotherapy used to have a dismal outcome. With the advent of low intensity combination treatment using hypomethylating agent and BCL2 inhibitor venetoclax, 30–40% of these patients can survive beyond 3 years. Supportive treatment at diagnosis and during the course of chemotherapy are essential to prevent complications. Platelet and packed cell transfusions are often needed. Fever should be managed promptly, and patients should be treated empirically with broad spectrum antibiotics. Fungal prophylaxis is also important as prolonged neutropenia is expected during induction chemotherapy.

8.10   KEY POINTS

1. AML is characterised by an abnormal increase in blasts of myeloid lineage in blood and/or BM.
2. Each AML shows distinct morphologic, cytochemical, immunophenotypic, cytogenetic and genetic features. When treated with standard induction and consolidation chemotherapy, patients show distinct responses and can be categorised into favourable, intermediate and adverse risk groups.
3. MRD plays an integral part in the management of AML and can be used to guide clinical treatment.

ADDITIONAL READING

1. Döhner H, Wei AH, Appelbaum FR et al. Diagnosis and management of AML in adults: 2022 recommendations from an international expert panel on behalf of the ELN. Blood 2022; 140(12): 1345–1377.

9 Acute Myeloid Leukaemia II

9.1 CLINICAL SCENARIO

A 76-year-old woman, with well controlled diabetes mellitus and hyperlipidaemia, has enjoyed independent activity of daily living. She presented with a 1-week history of malaise and shortness of breath on exertion. She was pale on physical examination.

9.2 LABORATORY REPORTS

	Results	References	Units
Haemoglobin	4.1	13–17	g/dL
Mean corpuscular volume	100.8	82–95.5	fL
White cell count	7.9	4–10	10^9/L
Platelet count	176	154–371	10^9/L

Blood film showed the presence of blasts at 49%. Auer rods were present (Figure 9.1A).

9.3 QUESTIONS

1. What is the diagnosis?
2. What are the further investigations?
3. What is the management plan?

9.4 PATIENT PROGRESS

Bone marrow (BM) aspiration showed the predominance of blasts (45%), which were strongly positive for myeloperoxidase (MPO). Cytogenetics showed normal karyotype. The blasts showed mutation of nucleophosmin 1 (*NPM1*). The patient received combination treatment of hypomethylating agent azacitidine and BCL2 inhibitor venetoclax. Reassessment BM after two cycles of treatment showed morphologic remission with count recovery. More importantly, minimal (measurable) residual disease (MRD) based on detection of *NPM1* mutation became negative after four cycles of treatment. Thereafter, she received continuous treatment with this combinaion as maintenance and has remained MRD negative for three years since first treatment. She has remained independent in her daily activities and has enjoyed travelling with her family.

9.5 ACUTE MYELOID LEUKAEMIA (AML)

Acute myeloid leukaemia (AML) is a group of diseases with diverse clinicopathologic, immunotypic, cytogenetic and genetic changes that share in common an abnormal increase in blasts in blood and BM. AML occurs in 3 patients per 100,000 every year, and its incidence has increased in recent decades. It occurs more commonly in the elderly population, with 60% of patients older than 65 years and a median age of 65 years. It is a highly lethal disease and is the fifth most deadly cancer, particularly in the elderly who are ineligible for standard treatment. About 50% of AML patients carry normal cytogenetics, and they show on average 2–4 recurrent mutations in different combinations, some of which are considered "drivers" and others "passengers" in leukaemogenesis.

DOI: 10.1201/9781003325413-11

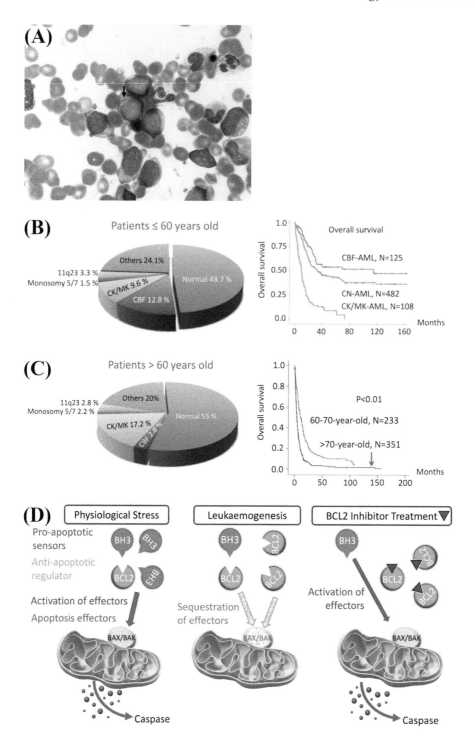

FIGURE 9.1 (A) Blood film showed the presence of blasts and Auer rods (arrow) (May-Grünwald Giemsa × 1000). (B,C) Distinct cytogenetic subtypes and overall survival in young (B) and elderly (C) patients with acute myeloid leukaemia. CBF: Core binding factor; CN: Cytogenetically normal; CK/MK: Complex or monosomy karyotype; AML: Acute myeloid leukaemia. (D) Pathogenetic role of BCL2 family in AML and the mechanism of action of BCL2 inhibitor.

In particular, *NPM1* mutation and bZIP in-frame mutation of *CEBPα* are associated with a favourable response to conventional chemotherapy, whereas *FLT3*-ITD is associated with a less favourable response. Approximately 10–15% of AML patients carry t(8;21) translocation (*RUNX1::RUNX1T1*) or inversion of chromosome 16 (*CBFβ::MYH11*), both of which involve components of core binding factor (CBF), which is a heterodimeric transcription factor comprising a non-DNA binding CBFβ chain and a DNA binding CBFα chain *RUNX1*. Another 10% of AML patients carry a complex (CK, ≥ 3 karyotypic abnormalities) or monosomy karyotype (MK, ≥ 2 monosomies or 1 monosomy and 1 structural abnormality), and this subtype portends an extremely poor prognosis. The rest of AML cases are made up of diverse diseases with different karyotypic and genetic abnormalities (Figure 9.1B). Elderly AML patients show a different spectrum of disease with higher prevalence of CK/MK AML and lower prevalence of CBF AML, which may account for an overall poor prognosis (Figure 9.1C).

9.6   TREATMENT OF ACUTE MYELOID LEUKAEMIA IN THE ELDERLY

In young and fit patients, induction and consolidation chemotherapy with or without allogeneic haematopoietic stem cell transplantation (HSCT) are the mainstays of treatment. Old and frail patients with AML show an extremely poor prognosis (Figure 9.1C). In addition to the aforementioned different disease spectrum, these patients are often ineligible for conventional treatment. Hypomethylating agents, including azacitidine and decitabine, have been shown to improve the overall survival of elderly AML patients, albeit modestly, but have little effects on the natural course of disease. More recently, the addition of BCL2 inhibitor venetoclax to hypomethylating agents has been shown to further improve patient survival. About 30–40% of patients can enjoy disease-free survival beyond 3 years, suggesting the possibility of a cure[1].

9.7   BCL2 INHIBITOR

BCL2 inhibitor venetoclax, in combination with hypomethylating agents, has changed the natural history of many elderly patients with AML and improved their clinical outcome (Figure 9.1D). The BCL2 family encompasses both pro-apoptotic and anti-apoptotic members. Apoptosis is a complex cellular process. It is accomplished by the activation and oligomerisation of effectors (e.g., BAX, BAK) in the mitochondrial membrane, leading to the release of apoptogenic proteins including cytochrome c. Under physiological conditions, apoptosis is prevented by the anti-apoptotic regulators including BCL2, MCL-1 and BCL-XL, which serve to sequester the effectors. In the presence of cellular stress, pro-apoptotic sensors (e.g., BIM, BID and PUMA) are activated, whose BH3 domain binds to the surface groove on the anti-apoptotic regulators and inhibits their regulatory function on the effectors. At the same time, the sensors can activate the effectors directly (Figure 9.1D). As a result, apoptosis ensues. Neoplastic cells including leukaemia blasts express excessive anti-apoptotic regulators, skewing the balance towards cellular survival. Venetoclax is a BH3 mimetic that binds specifically to the surface groove on BCL2 protein to block its interaction with the sensors. The sensors then become free to activate the pro-apoptotic effector, leading to apoptosis[2].

9.8   KEY POINTS

1. AML is more common in the elderly, in whom the disease subtypes are less chemo-responsive, and the patients are generally unfit, which accounts for the dismal outcomes.
2. A combination of hypomethylating agent and BCL2 inhibitor might induce long-term remission in elderly patients while preserving their quality of life.

ADDITIONAL READINGS

1. DiNardo CD, Jonas BA, Pullarkat V et al. Azacitidine and venetoclax in previously untreated acute myeloid leukaemia. New Engl J Med 2020; 383(7): 617–629.
2. Ashkenazi V, Fairbrother WJ, Leverson JD, Souers AJ. From basic apoptosis discoveries to advanced selective BCL-2 family inhibitors. Nat Rev Drug Dis 2017; 16: 273–284.

10 Myelodysplastic Syndrome

10.1 CLINICAL SCENARIO

A 49-year-old man had an annual check-up by his family physician. He was married and had 4 children. His mother died of lymphoma. He was a hepatitis B carrier on regular surveillance. He was known to have a somewhat high mean corpuscular volume (MCV) since 2016, but other blood parameters were normal. In 2019, his haemoglobin was 11.5 g/dL, MCV was 107 fL, white cell count was 3.2×10^9/L and platelet count was 242×10^9/L. He presented again with worsening blood counts in 2021.

10.2 LABORATORY REPORTS

	Results	Reference Range	Units
Haemoglobin	8.2	11.5–14.8	g/dL
MCV	106	82.0–95.5	fL
White cell count	2.2	3.89–9.93	10^9/L
Platelet count	80	167–396	10^9/L

Blood film showed occasional hypogranular and hypolobated neutrophils with normal differential count (Figure 10.1A).

10.3 QUESTIONS

1. What further investigations should be performed?
2. What is the likely diagnosis?
3. What is the management plan?

10.4 PROGRESS

Bone marrow (BM) examination showed hypercellularity and blasts that accounted for 8%. Erythroid precursors showed nuclear irregularity, and small hypolobated megakaryocytes were encountered (Figure 10.1A). Ring sideroblasts accounted for 27% of the erythroid precursors. A diagnosis of myelodysplastic syndrome with excess blasts (MDS-EB1) was made. Cytogenetics were 46, XY, and next generation sequencing (NGS) showed the presence of *SF3B1*, *ETNK1* and *KRAS* mutations.

The patient was treated with hypomethylating agent azacitidine. Despite an initial response for three months, he became dependent on red cell and platelet transfusions thereafter. A repeat BM examination showed a markedly hypercellular marrow, focal prominence of blasts (5–10%), active but dysplastic erythropoiesis and increased number of small and hypolobated megakaryocytes.

10.5 FURTHER QUESTION

1. What is the next management?

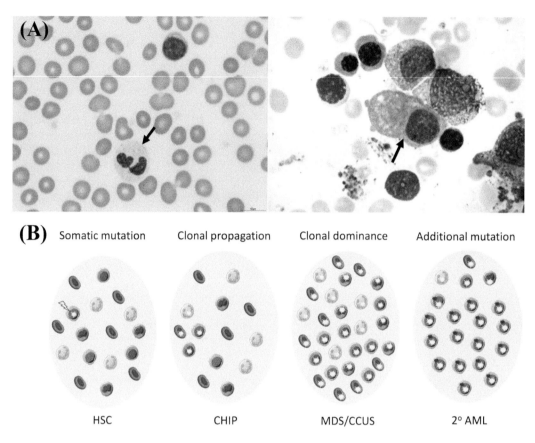

FIGURE 10.1 (A) Left: A hypolobated and hypogranular neutrophil (arrow) in myelodysplastic syndrome (MDS) (Wright-Giemsa × 1000). Right: Small hypolobulated megakaryocyte (or micromegakaryocyte) (arrow) in myelodysplastic syndrome. (B) Pathogenesis of MDS involves four distinct stages. HSC: Haematopoietic stem cell; CHIP: Clonal haematopoiesis of indeterminate potential; CCUS: Clonal cytopenia of unknown significance; AML: Acute myeloid leukaemia.

10.6 PROGRESS

The patient was referred for allogeneic haematopoietic stem cell transplantation (HSCT) from his son. He developed cytokine release syndrome on Day 1 of HSC infusion, when he presented with high fever and desaturation requiring supplemental oxygen. He received two doses of tocilizumab, and his symptoms subsided. He engrafted successfully on Day 19 of HSCT with the normalisation of blood counts.

10.7 MYELODYSPLASTIC SYNDROME

Myelodysplastic syndrome (MDS) occurs mainly in elderly patients with a median age of diagnosis of 70 years. Most patients present with persistent and unexplained cytopenia in one or more blood lineages, macrocytosis and dysplasia (Greek: *dys*—abnormal; *plasis*—formation) of the neutrophils, typically hypogranular cytoplasm and hypolobated nuclei, with or without circulating blasts. BM examination is essential, which characteristically shows hypercellularity with dysplasia, and underscores ineffective haematopoiesis. Morphological classification of MDS is based on the number of blood lineages showing cytopenia in peripheral blood and dysplasia in BM, the percentage of ring sideroblasts and the percentage of blasts in blood and BM. Cytogenetic abnormalities in MDS are diverse. Different abnormalities are associated with distinct prognoses, and together with the extent of cytopenia and BM blasts, constitute the revised International Prognostic Scoring System (IPSS-R). More recently, somatic mutations are incorporated into the prognostication of MDS to form the R-IPSS-M. Mutations of genes encoding for *SF3B1*, *TET2*, *SRSF2*, *ASXL1*, *DNMT3A* and *RUNX1* occur in at least 10% of MDS patients. At diagnosis, the median number of driver mutations is 2–3. In the past, an arbitrary cut-off of 20% blood or BM blasts was adopted to distinguish between MDS (< 20%) and acute myeloid leukaemia (AML) (≥ 20%). In 2022, the International Consensus Classification recognised MDS and AML as a continuum and cases with 10–20% blasts in blood or BM are classified as MDS/AML.

10.8 PATHOGENESIS

With the advances in genomic sequencing, it is becoming clear that the pathogenesis of full-blown MDS involves distinct stages, culminating in the transformation into AML (Figure 10.1B). The **first phase** begins with somatic mutation of an HSC that confers proliferative and survival advantage, which generates a clone of mutated HSC and its progenies. The **second phase** is characterised by propagation of the mutant clone, known as clonal haematopoiesis of indeterminate potential (CHIP), which is detectable in blood by the presence of somatic mutations in circulating leukocytes. The predominant CHIP mutations occur in genes associated with epigenetic regulation, *viz.*, *DNMT3A*, *TET2* or *ASXL1*, and spliceosome function, *viz.*, *SF3B1*, *SRSF2* or *U2AF1*. The **third phase** is characterised by the expansion of clones some of which become dominant. Clinically, clonal dominance is associated with MDS or clonal cytopenia of undetermined significance (CCUS). The **fourth phase** is characterised by the selection of clones, which is often associated with the acquisition of additional driver mutations that cause differentiation blockades or increased proliferation, culminating in leukaemic transformation.

10.9 DIFFERENTIAL DIAGNOSIS

A thorough drug history is important to ascertain drug-related dysplastic BM changes, including the use of isoniazid and alcohol intake, which may induce ring sideroblast formation; antibiotic cotrimoxazole, immunosuppression tacrolimus and mycophenolate mofetil, which may cause neutrophil hyposegmentation; and granulocyte colony-stimulating factor (G-CSF) injection, which may cause an increase in blasts. Nutritional causes of marrow dysplasia should also be considered, including vitamin B12, copper or zinc deficiency.

10.10 TREATMENT

Treatment of MDS is determined by factors pertaining to disease prognostication and the fitness of patients. **Treatment of low-risk MDS** aims at quality of life improvement and reduction of transfusion dependence and infective complications. This entails growth factor support with G-CSF and erythropoiesis-stimulating agents (ESA), with ESA being more effective in patients with serum erythropoietin of less than 400 U/L. In addition, treatments are available for patients with specific MDS subtypes including lenalidomide for those with del(5q) and luspatercept for those with MDS with ring sideroblasts. **In patients with high-risk MDS**, hypomethylating agents, *viz.*, azacitidine or decitabine, are the mainstays of treatment. In elderly and unfit patients, treatment should be continued until progression or a lack of response after at least 4 courses as delayed responses may occur. More recently, the addition of BCL2 inhibitor venetoclax, which is used for the treatment of elderly AML, has also been shown to be effective in MDS. In young and fit patients, allogeneic HSCT should be considered for curative treatment.

10.11   KEY POINTS

1. MDS is characterised by peripheral cytopenia, marrow hypercellularity and morphological dysplasia, underscoring ineffective haematopoiesis.
2. MDS pathogenesis involves distinct stages, beginning from somatic mutations of HSC to clonal propagation and dominance and finally, transformation into AML.
3. Management of low-risk MDS is about reducing transfusions and complications and preserving the quality of life. Management of high-risk disease involves mitigating its natural progression in elderly patients and disease eradication by allogeneic HSCT in young and fit patients.

ADDITIONAL READING

1. Cazzola M. Myelodysplastic syndromes. N Engl J Med 2020; 383(14): 1358–1374.

11 Chronic Myeloid Leukaemia

11.1 CLINICAL SCENARIO

A 52-year-old man, who is a chronic smoker with a history of coronary artery disease and percutaneous coronary intervention (PCI) 10 years ago, presented with left upper abdomen discomfort, weight loss of 15 pounds (baseline body weight 140 pounds) and night sweats over 3 months. His mother died of lung cancer at age 60 years. Physical examination showed splenomegaly of 8 cm below the costal margin.

11.2 LABORATORY REPORTS

	Results	References	Units
Haemoglobin	10.7	13.3–17.1	g/dL
White cell count	211.47	3.89–9.92	10^9/L
Platelet count	307	154–371	10^9/L

Liver and renal function tests: Unremarkable.

Blood smear showed a leukoerythroblastic blood picture. Neutrophils and myelocytes accounted for 46 and 34%, respectively. Basophils and blasts accounted for 7 and 2%, respectively (Figure 11.1A). Bone marrow aspirate showed marked hypercellularity. Granulopoiesis was markedly increased with the bimodal prominence of myelocytes and neutrophils. Blasts were not increased, and basophilia and eosinophilia were seen. Megakaryopoiesis was increased with the prominence of a small and hypolobated form (Figure 11.1B).

11.3 QUESTIONS

1. What is the diagnosis?
2. What other investigations are needed?
3. What is the management plan?

11.4 CLINICAL PROGRESS

The morphologic diagnosis was chronic myeloid leukaemia in the chronic phase (CML-CP). Cytogenetic and fluorescence in-situ hybridisation (FISH) analyses confirmed both t(9;22) and *BCR::ABL1* fusion (Figures 11.1C and 11.1D). Reverse transcription polymerase chain reaction (RT-PCR) detected the presence of e14a2 *BCR::ABL1* transcript. The patient was treated with first generation tyrosine kinase inhibitor (TKI) imatinib. Except for oedema over the legs and scrotum and thrombocytopenia, he tolerated the treatment well. After 5 years of treatment, he achieved deep molecular response with a 5-log reduction of transcripts (Figure 11.2A).

11.5 PATHOGENESIS

Chronic myeloid leukaemia (CML) is characterised by the presence of Philadelphia chromosome t(9;22), the resulting *BCR::ABL1* fusion gene and constitutive activation of the tyrosine kinase ABL1

DOI: 10.1201/9781003325413-13

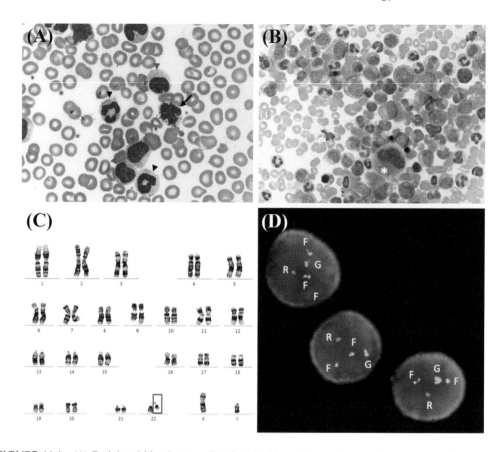

FIGURE 11.1 (A) Peripheral blood smear showing the bimodal prominence of neutrophils (black arrowheads) and myelocytes (red arrowheads), in association with basophilia (arrow). (Wright-Giemsa × 1000). (B) Bone marrow aspirate showing granulocytic hyperplasia due to the bimodal prominence of neutrophils and myelocytes. Erythroid activity is depressed, and a small hypolobulated megakaryocyte (asterisk) is found. (Wright-Giemsa × 400). (C) Karyotype showing 46,XY,t(9;22)(q34;q11). G-banding by trypsin/Giemsa. The red box indicates the Philadelphia chromosome. (D): Interphase fluorescence in-situ hybridisation by Dual Colour Dual Fusion BCR::ABL1 probe, showing a 2F1R1G positive signal pattern in the three cells. R: Red; G: Green; F: Fusion.

(Figures 11.2B–11.2D). The breakpoint in chromosome 9 occurs consistently between exons 1 and 2, whereas the breakpoint in chromosome 22 occurs in various locations at the major breakpoint region. The variable breakpoints produce two distinct transcripts, specifically, e13a2 (formerly b2a2) and e14a2 (formerly b3a2), which both generate a BCR::ABL1 protein of 210 kDa molecular weight. Occasionally, the breakpoint occurs at the minor breakpoint region and generates an e1a2 transcript that translates into a BCR::ABL1 protein of 190 kDa. A rare isoform of the BCR::ABL1 protein of 230 kDa also exists.

11.6   CLINICAL PRESENTATION

Some patients may present with incidental findings of abnormal blood tests during check-up and may be entirely asymptomatic. Other patients may present with left upper quadrant discomfort and early satiety due to splenomegaly or constitutional symptoms, including fever, weight loss and night sweats. Occasionally, patients may present with symptoms of leukostasis including headaches, visual disturbance, shortness of breath or priapism. Patients who present at blastic crisis may have symptoms of acute leukaemia, including bleeding, anaemia and fever due to infections.

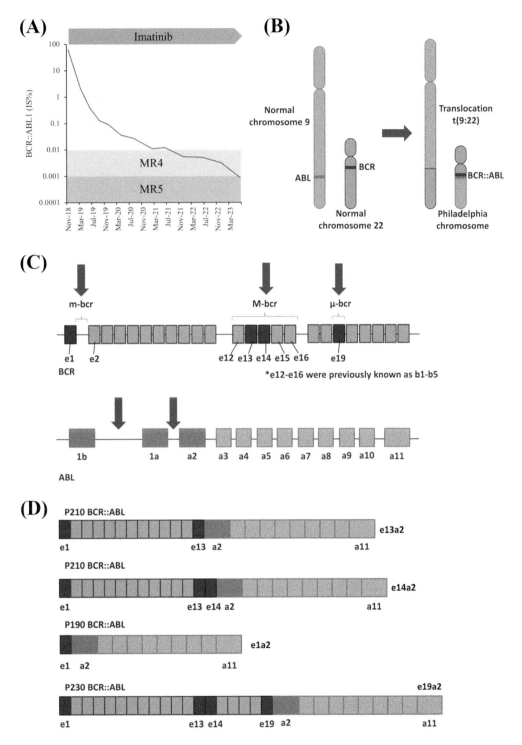

FIGURE 11.2 (A): Minimal (measurable) residual disease (MRD) monitoring based on *BCR::ABL1* from peripheral blood. MR: Molecular response. MR4 and 5 refer to 4 and 5-log reduction, respectively. They are defined as deep molecular response. (B): Normal structure of chromosome 9 and 22 and the formation of a Philadelphia chromosome. (C): Molecular structures of *BCR* and *ABL1* and the breakpoints (arrows). (D): Molecular structures of various *BCR-ABL1* fusions. (*Figure 11.2A, courtesy of Dr. Carol Cheung.*)

11.7   LABORATORY DIAGNOSIS

The initial clue to the diagnosis of CML is usually leukocytosis with a typical bimodal distribution, i.e., predominant neutrophils and myelocytes. Absolute basophil and eosinophil counts may be raised, and thrombocytosis is common. Bone marrow features are characteristic. Demonstration of the pathognomonic Philadelphia chromosome is essential, and this can be achieved by conventional karyotyping showing t(9;22) translocation, FISH or RT-PCR showing the *BCR::ABL1* fusion gene. Quantification of the *BCR::ABL1* fusion gene is also essential as a baseline based on which subsequent treatment response to TKI can be evaluated.

11.8   PROGNOSTIC FACTORS

A number of prognostic scores (Sokal, Hasford and EUTOS scores) have been developed to predict the treatment outcome of patients and the risk of disease progression based on clinical parameters at diagnosis, including patient age, spleen size and haematological indexes (platelet, basophil, eosinophil and blast counts).

11.9   NATURAL DISEASE COURSE

CML progression entails two distinct phases, namely, chronic phase (CP) and blastic crisis (BC), which could be lymphoblastic or myeloblastic. There is also an intermediate accelerated phase (AP). Most CML patients present at CP. In the pre-TKI era, CP patients ineligible for haematopoietic stem cell transplantation (HSCT) would progress to BC in a median of 3 years. Once transformed to BC, median survival is approximately 6 months. TKI is now the mainstay of treatment for CML-CP, and disease progression is infrequently seen. Occasionally, CML patients may present as AP or even BC.

11.10   MANAGEMENT OF CML

CML has been a foundational model in which the identification of a single driving event, i.e., *BCR::ABL1*, resulted in the development of the **first generation** TKI imatinib, which was tested in randomised controlled trials with proven survival benefit over interferon and cytarabine, as these were the standard management then. Generic imatinib is now available and leads to a substantial reduction in cost and much better affordability. **Second generation** TKI (dasatinib, nilotinib and bosutinib) has been developed for use in some patients who developed resistance or were intolerant to imatinib. A major consideration in the management of CML has been the emergence of the Thr315Ile mutation in *BCR::ABL1*, which is resistant to first and second generation TKI. This led to the development of ponatinib, a **third generation** TKI effective against Thr315Ile mutation. Asciminib, a **fourth generation** TKI that binds the myristoyl- rather than ATP-binding pocket of ABL1, was recently approved for CML-CP failing ≥ 2 prior TKI. A number of clinical trials comparing second generation TKI with imatinib in the first-line treatment of CML showed superior efficacy in inducing molecular response, leading to their approval for this indication. However, this superior efficacy has not resulted in better overall or progression-free survival in these studies. The decision on the choice of first versus second generation TKI for upfront treatment of CML-CP should be individualised. Allogeneic HSCT, once the standard of care for CML-CP, is now rarely performed for CML except for patients with progression or those who present at CML-BC.

11.11   MONITORING TREATMENT RESPONSE TO TKI

With the favourable efficacy of TKI, a major consideration in patient management is about disease monitoring so that early intervention is possible. Emerging evidence shows the possibility of treatment cessation in patients who could achieve sustained complete molecular remission. In the past, treatment response was assessed based on detection of CML clone size using cytogenetic analysis, fluorescence in-situ hybridisation and quantitative PCR (qPCR). Currently, qPCR has become the standard of care by virtue of its sensitivity, automation and rapid throughput. At present, a deep molecular response MR4·5 (i.e., *BCR::ABL1* ≤ 0·0032% as measured on the International Scale) is considered the treatment goal for practical purposes. A number of clinical trials are evaluating the possibility of treatment cessation and achievement of treatment-free remission.

11.12   KEY POINTS

1. CML-CP is characterised by leukocytosis with a prominence of neutrophils and myelocytes and the presence of t(9;22) translocation that results in *BCR::ABL1* fusion and constitutive activation of tyrosine kinase ABL1.
2. TKI against *BCR::ABL1* is the mainstay of treatment. The first generation imatinib is the prototype, which shows survival benefits over conventional treatment.
3. The monitoring of treatment response based on *BCR::ABL1* detection is key to the management of CML.

ADDITIONAL READING

1. Cortes J, Pavlovsky C, Saußele S. Chronic myeloid leukaemia. Lancet 2021; 398(10314): 1914–1926.

12 Essential Thrombocytosis

12.1 CLINICAL SCENARIO

A 41-year-old woman with good past health had blood tests before planning for pregnancy. She was otherwise asymptomatic. She was married with no children. There was no family history of blood diseases or malignancies. Physical examination was unremarkable.

12.2 LABORATORY REPORTS

	Results	Reference Range	Units
Haemoglobin	12.0	11.5–14.8	g/dL
Mean corpuscular volume	95	82.0–95.5	fL
White cell count	5.0	3.89–9.93	10^9/L
Platelet count	920	167–396	10^9/L

Blood smear showed thrombocytosis with no abnormal red cell or white cell morphology (Figure 12.1A).

Liver and renal function tests and lactate dehydrogenase: Normal

12.3 QUESTIONS

1. What additional investigations should be performed?
2. What is the likely diagnosis?
3. What is the management plan?

12.4 CLINICAL PROGRESS

The patient's serum iron, total iron binding capacity and transferrin saturation were within normal limits. Immune markers including anti-nuclear antibody, rheumatoid factor, C-reactive protein and tumour markers were all negative. Bone marrow aspiration (Figure 12.1B) and biopsy (Figure 12.1C) were performed, which showed features of myeloproliferative neoplasm; this favours essential thrombocytosis. Cytogenetics were normal. Next generation sequencing (NGS) showed calreticulin exon 9 mutation (Figure 12.1D) as the only abnormality. A diagnosis of essential thrombocytosis (ET) was made. The patient was given aspirin and PEGylated interferon 2α injections, and her platelet count became normal. She became pregnant thereafter while continuing the treatment and had a normal delivery.

12.5 DIFFERENTIAL DIAGNOSIS AND CLINICAL PRESENTATION

In patients with thrombocytosis, secondary causes, including iron deficiency anaemia, infection, post-surgical or trauma state or malignancy, should be excluded. However, certain clinical features are suggestive of ET. The median age of onset of ET is 60 years, and there is a slight female preponderance. Patients may present with an incidental finding of thrombocytosis or with symptoms such as recurrent headache, visual disturbance, light-headedness, dysaesthesia (abnormal sense of touch)

DOI: 10.1201/9781003325413-14

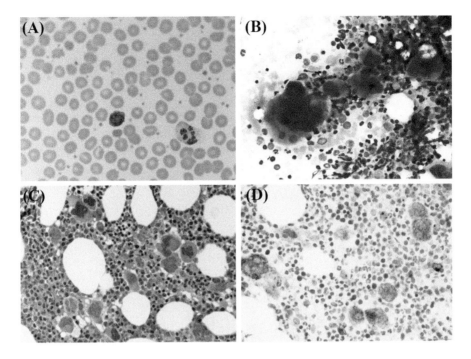

FIGURE 12.1   (A) Blood smear of the patient showing thrombocytosis (Wright-Giemsa × 1000). (B) Bone marrow aspirate showing increased pleomorphic megakaryocytes that include large and hyperlobulated forms (Wight-Giemsa × 1000). (C) Trephine biopsy showing hyperplastic bone marrow and marked megakaryocytic hyperplasia (H&E × 400). (D) The presence of CALR mutation in megakaryocytes can be detected by immunohistochemistry based on antibody detection of a novel elongated C-terminal peptide arising from the mutation (× 400).

or erythromelalgia (painful swelling and redness of extremities). Thrombosis at or before diagnosis occurs in about 20% of patients. On examination, palpable splenomegaly may occur.

Myeloproliferative neoplasms including ET, primary myelofibrosis (early or pre-fibrotic variant), polycythaemia vera (PV) and chronic myeloid leukaemia (CML) are associated with thrombocytosis. Although the presence of polycythaemia and Philadelphia chromosome would readily lead to the diagnoses of PV and CML, distinction between ET and early or pre-fibrotic primary myelofibrosis could be challenging. Such distinction is clinically relevant as primary myelofibrosis is associated with a lower patient survival, higher risk of leukaemic transformation and progression of myelofibrosis. In addition to the characteristic pathologic features in bone marrow, normal haemoglobin and serum lactate dehydrogenase, the absence of leukoerythroblastic blood picture or tear-drop cells would suggest a diagnosis of ET.

12.6   GENETICS OF ESSENTIAL THROMBOCYTOSIS

With the advances of NGS, the mutation landscape of ET has become clear. Mutations of genes encoding for janus kinase 2 (JAK2), calreticulin (CALR) and myeloproliferative leukemia (MPL) protein are considered driver mutations. In contrast to PV, in which *JAK2* mutation occurs in over 95% of patients, only 60% of ET patients carry this mutation. Mutations of genes encoding for CALR and MPL occur in approximately 20 and 3% of patients, respectively, and triple negative conditions occur in about 10–20% of patients. Non-driver mutations also occur in ET and include *ASXL1, EZH2, TET2, IDH1, IDH2, SRSF2* and *SF3B1*. In clinical practice, the presence of these mutations substantiates the diagnosis of myeloproliferative neoplasm (MPN) particularly in the triple negative cases.

12.7 COMPLICATIONS OF ESSENTIAL THROMBOCYTOSIS

Thrombosis, either arterial or venous, is a major complication in ET. The four major risk factors for thrombosis in ET include age (> 60 years old), prior thrombotic episodes, coexisting cardiovascular risk factors and the presence of the *JAK2*V617F mutation. These risk factors impact the indication of antiplatelet agents and cytoreduction therapy (see the following). In contrast, extreme thrombocytosis (Platelet count > 1000×10^9/L) is associated with acquired Von Willebrand Disease and bleeding risk due to adsorption of Von Willebrand multimers on the platelet surface.

12.8 PROGNOSIS

In general, ET patients have slightly shorter survival than the general population, but they show the most favourable survival among other MPN. An important consideration in predicting the prognosis of ET patients is the distinction from pre-fibrotic myelofibrosis as previously mentioned. In patients with *bona fide* ET, a number of clinical and genetic factors are predictive of patient survival. These include age, the presence of leukocytosis, a history of thrombosis and the presence of specific mutations of *SRSF2*, *U2AF1*, *SF3B1* or *TP53*. A number of prognosis calculators that incorporate these factors are available online.

12.9 TREATMENT

Treatment of ET depends on the risk of thrombosis, which is the major cause of morbidity. Patients with low risk can be managed with observation or low-dose aspirin. Those with high-risk disease should be given additional cytoreduction therapy, which currently includes hydroxyurea, interferon or anagrelide. In general, hydroxyurea is the first-line cytoreduction therapy, which is associated with relatively low toxicity. Anagrelide, which selectively inhibits megakaryocyte differentiation and reduces thrombocytosis, can also be used, although data have conflicted with respect to its benefit and safety compared with hydroxyurea. PEGylated interferon is effective for ET and may reduce neoplastic clones in some patients. However, it requires subcutaneous injection and may be associated with more side effects including deranged liver function and depression. It is particularly useful in conditions in which hydroxyurea is contraindicated or should be avoided, such as young patients (< 40 years old), women of childbearing age or patients who are diagnosed with ET during pregnancy. Histologically, radioactive phosphorous P32 or alkylators such as chlorambucil have been used but are associated with a significant risk of secondary leukaemia.

12.10 KEY POINTS

1. In patients with thrombocytosis, secondary causes should always be considered first.
2. The major complication of ET is thrombosis, which can be arterial or venous.
3. Treatment of ET should aim at reducing the risk of thrombosis. It includes aspirin and hydroxyurea. PEGylated interferon can be considered in young patients and in women of childbearing age or during pregnancy.

ADDITIONAL READINGS

1. Tefferi A, Pardanani A. Essential thrombocythemia. N Engl J Med 2019; 381: 2135–2144.
2. Stein H, Bob R, Durkop H et al. A new monoclonal antibody (CAL2) detects CALRETICULIN mutations in formalin-fixed and paraffin-embedded bone marrow biopsies. Leukemia 2016; 30: 131–135.

13 Polycythaemia Vera

13.1 CLINICAL SCENARIO

A 74-year-old woman, who was a non-smoker, was found to have raised haemoglobin during a health check-up in 2013. She was plethoric, and abdominal examination showed a palpable spleen tip.

13.2 LABORATORY REPORTS IN 2013

	Results	Reference Range	Units
Haemoglobin	20.1	11.5–14.8	g/dL
Haematocrit	0.65	0.36–0.48	fL
White cell count	10.3	3.89–9.93	10^9/L
Platelet count	401	167–396	10^9/L
Serum erythropoietin	3.16	2.2–19.0	mIU/mL

Blood smear showed increases in red cell, neutrophil and platelet counts (Figure 13.1A). Bone marrow showed increased cellularity and trilineage hyperplasia. Megakaryocytes were increased in number and occurred in clusters. They were pleomorphic, and some were large and hyperlobulated. Stainable iron was absent (Figure 13.1B). *JAK2*V617 mutation was detected.

13.3 QUESTIONS

1. What is the likely diagnosis?
2. What is the management plan?
3. What is the prognosis?

13.4 CLINICAL PROGRESS

A diagnosis of polycythaemia vera (PV) was made. The patient underwent regular venesection at bimonthly intervals and received aspirin and hydroxyurea. Her blood counts have been stable with haemoglobin around 15–16 g/dL and haematocrit around 0.4. She became progressively anaemic in 2020 even after cessation of venesection and hydroxyurea. She had low-grade fever and significant weight loss. Abdominal examination showed hepatosplenomegaly about 2–3 fingerbreadths below the costal margin.

13.5 LABORATORY REPORTS IN 2021

Haemoglobin: 6.6 g/dL, frequent tear-drop cells and nucleated RBC. Little polychromasia.
White cell count: 6.9×10^9/L, presence of myelocytes and blasts (1%)
Platelet count: 17×10^9/L

Bone marrow (BM) showed marked hypercellularity. Megakaryocytic hyperplasia was seen with size heterogeneity and abnormal topographical distribution. Reticulin fibres were diffusely coarsened. Next generation sequencing showed in addition to *JAK2*V617F, the presence of a *TP53* mutation.

DOI: 10.1201/9781003325413-15

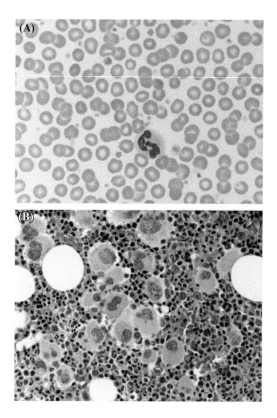

FIGURE 13.1   (A) Peripheral blood smear of a polycythaemia vera (PV) patient showing a packed smear due to increased red cell and platelet counts (Wright-Giemsa × 1000). (B) Bone marrow of a PV patient showing marked megakaryocytic hyperplasia and pleomorphism, in association with erythroid hyperplasia (H&E × 400).

She received a course of thalidomide and prednisolone for her anaemia with little effects and became transfusion-dependent. She also received ruxolitinib with some improvement in constitutional symptoms. Her condition deteriorated thereafter, and she succumbed to an episode of intracranial haemorrhage.

13.6   CLINICAL FEATURES

In patients with an abnormal increase in haemoglobin, secondary causes of polycythaemia, which are frequently due to chronic hypoxaemia secondary to smoking and respiratory diseases including obstructive sleep apnoea, chronic obstructive airway diseases or bronchiectasis, should be ruled out. Rarely, solid cancers such as hepatocellular or renal cell carcinoma or brain tumour may give rise to polycythaemia.

Polycythaemia vera (PV) belongs to the family of myeloproliferative neoplasm (MPN) and is characterised by excessive production of erythrocytes. It is defined by i) an increase in haemoglobin or haematocrit; ii) the presence of *JAK2*V617 or exon 12 mutation; iii) characteristic BM morphology; and iv) a subnormal level of serum erythropoietin. The first two criteria are essential, whereas only one of the remaining two criteria is needed for diagnostic purposes. PV is the most common MPN with a median age of onset of about 60 years. Patients may be asymptomatic or may present with generalised pruritus, erythromelalgia (i.e., painful redness and swelling of extremities due to red cells and platelet aggregation in blood vessels) or symptoms related to splenomegaly.

13.7 PROGNOSIS

In general, the overall survival of PV patient is inferior to that of the age- and sex-matched general population. Factors predictive of prognosis include age, leukocytosis, venous thrombosis and abnormal karyotype. More recently, specific gene mutations, *viz.*, *SRSF2*, *IDH2*, *RUNX1* and *U2AF1*, are shown to confer an adverse prognosis on PV patients. Prognosis calculators incorporating these factors are available online. Post-PV myelofibrosis is a major factor leading to mortality in PV patients, and when this happens, prognosis is often predicted based on the clinicopathologic parameters used for primary myelofibrosis (e.g., DIPSS Plus online). More recently, mutation-enhanced prognostic models are available that take into consideration specific high-risk mutations, e.g., *ASXL1*, *SRSF2*, *EZH2* or *IDH1/IDH2*, or the lack of favourable mutations, e.g., calreticulin (*CALR*).

13.8 COMPLICATIONS

Arterial or venous thrombosis is a major complication in PV patients. The risk of thrombosis increases with age, leukocytosis, *JAK2*V617 allelic burden, previous episodes of thrombosis and for arterial thrombosis, coexisting cardiovascular risk factors.

13.9 MANAGEMENT PLAN

Regular phlebotomy and aspirin are the mainstays of treatment for all patients with PV. The treatment goal of phlebotomy is to maintain haematocrit < 0.45 and reduce risks of thrombotic and cardiovascular events. Cytoreduction is needed for the control of disease-related symptoms, e.g., pruritus and splenomegaly. Hydroxyurea is the treatment of choice for older patients. PEGylated interferon should be considered for younger patients, female patients of childbearing age and during pregnancy. For patients who are intolerant or refractory to hydroxyurea, PEGylated interferon or ruxolitinib (a JAK 1/2 inhibitor) should be used. Previous treatments including chlorambucil and radioactive phosphorous P32 are largely obsolete because of their leukaemogenic potential. Younger patients with post-PV myelofibrosis should be considered for allogeneic haematopoietic stem cell transplantation (HSCT).

13.10 KEY POINTS

1. Secondary causes of polycythaemia should be considered in patients with raised haemoglobin.
2. *JAK2*V617 or exon 12 mutation occurs in > 99% of PV patients and is essential for diagnosis.
3. Phlebotomy, aspirin and cytoreduction are the mainstays of treatment.
4. Post-PV myelofibrosis is a major factor leading to mortality in PV patients.

ADDITIONAL READING

1. Tefferi A, Vannucchi AM, Barbui T. Polycythemia vera: historical oversights, diagnostic details and therapeutic views. Leukemia 2021; 35: 3339–3351.

14 Primary Myelofibrosis

14.1 CLINICAL SCENARIO

A 68-year-old man who had Diabetes mellitus (DM) and atrial flutter presented with progressive malaise, weight loss, poor appetite and early satiety for one year. He was emaciated, and his spleen was palpable, measuring 4 fingerbreadths below the costal margin.

14.2 LABORATORY REPORTS

	Results	Reference Range	Units
Haemoglobin	6.0	11.5–14.8	g/dL
White cell count	1.7	3.89–9.93	10^9/L
Platelet count	361	167–396	10^9/L
Lactate dehydrogenase	601	120–220	IU/L

Liver and renal function tests: Unremarkable.
Blood smear: Leukoerythroblastic blood picture; presence of tear-drop cells.

Bone marrow was hypercellular for age. Megakaryocytes were increased and showed increased pleomorphism, with some showing hyperlobulated nuclei and others showing pyknotic nuclei. Blasts were focally prominent. Reticular fibres were diffusely coarsened (Figure 14.1). Cytogenetic analysis showed deletion of chromosome 13q34. *JAK2*V617 mutation was detectable.

14.3 QUESTIONS

1. What is the likely diagnosis?
2. What is the management plan?
3. What is the prognosis?

14.4 CLINICAL PROGRESS

The patient was given 10 units of blood transfusion in less than 6 months and began to receive ruxolitinib. Within 1 month of treatment, the spleen became impalpable, and early satiety had also improved. His body weight increased from 52.8 to 55.7 kg. He remained transfusion-dependent, requiring blood transfusion once every 2–4 weeks. Three years later, he experienced weight loss again, and a spleen tip became palpable. Bone marrow examination showed an increase in blast counts of up to 23%. In addition to *JAK2* mutation, *ASXL1* mutation was detected. His condition deteriorated rapidly, and he succumbed to an episode of COVID-19 infection.

14.5 CLINICAL PRESENTATION

Primary myelofibrosis is mainly a disease of the elderly with a median age of onset at about 65 years old. In most cases, patients present with anaemia, bone and abdominal pain, early satiety, constitutional symptoms and pruritus. Hepatosplenomegaly can be marked. In severe cases, portal hypertension may occur, leading to variceal bleeding and ascites. Aberrant cytokine release from neoplastic

 DOI: 10.1201/9781003325413-16

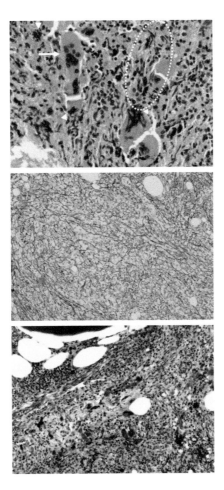

FIGURE 14.1 (Upper) Trephine biopsy features the streaming of haemopoietic cells (dotted lines) due to stromal fibrosis and large hyperlobulated megakaryocytes (arrow) that show increased nuclear pyknosis (arrowhead) (H&E × 400). (Middle) Diffuse coarsening of the reticulin fibres that show numerous intersections. (Lower) Extensive interstitial collagen fibrosis as detected by the trichrome stain.

cells and the host immune reaction may result in constitutional symptoms and cachexia, which are the major causes of morbidity. Causes of mortality include leukaemic transformation, which occurs in up to 30% of cases; opportunistic infection and bleeding due to neutropenia and thrombocytopenia; and cardiovascular events including arterial thrombosis and pulmonary embolism.

14.6 DIAGNOSIS

Diagnosis of primary myelofibrosis (PMF) depends on the detection of characteristic clinical and laboratory features and the **exclusion of other myeloproliferative neoplasms**. The presence of anaemia, constitutional symptoms and splenomegaly are typical presentations. Careful examination of **blood smear** is needed to ascertain the presence of the leukoerythroblastic blood picture and teardrop red cells. Lactate dehydrogenase (LDH) is characteristically raised. Bone marrow examination is essential for the detection of abnormal megakaryocyte proliferation and morphology and the severity of reticulin fibrosis, and the latter may distinguish the early/pre-fibrotic stage from overtly fibrotic PMF. Cytogenetic analysis is essential to rule out the presence of Philadelphia chromosome, which is pathognomonic of chronic myeloid leukaemia and to detect the characteristic karyotype of PMF, including +9, del(13q), del(20q) and 1q duplication. Genetic analysis is also essential, and PMF is associated with driver mutations including *JAK2*, *CALR* or *MPL* mutation, and mutations of *ASXL1*, *SRSF2*, *U2AF1*, *EZH2* and *IDH1/2* are associated with adverse prognosis. An important differential diagnosis of pre-fibrotic PMF is essential thrombocytosis, and the latter can be distinguished by the morphological features and topographical distribution of megakaryocytes, the lack of leukoerythroblastic pictures, the absence of tear-drop red cells and normal LDH. A diagnosis of myelodysplastic syndrome (MDS) or MDS/myeloproliferative neoplasm (MPN) should be considered in the presence of dyserythropoiesis or dysgranulopoiesis, particularly in the absence of driver mutations for PMF. Acute megakaryoblastic leukaemia and primary autoimmune myelofibrosis are rare entities that may mimic PMF.

14.7 PROGNOSTICATION

Prediction of the outcome of PMF at diagnosis and any timepoint thereafter, with particular reference to the risk of leukaemic transformation and survival, is important for the consideration of allogeneic haematopoietic stem cell transplantation (HSCT) for eligible patients. A number of clinicopathologic features are predictive of outcome, including **age**, the presence of **constitutional symptoms**, **haemoglobin**, **leukocyte counts** and **circulating blasts**. These features at diagnosis were incorporated in the International Prognostic Scoring System (IPSS), and those examined at subsequent timepoints were incorporated in the Dynamic IPSS. Additional features including **thrombocytopenia**, the need for **red cell transfusion** and the presence of **unfavourable karyotype** were incorporated in the DIPSS Plus. New prognostic models have emerged that incorporate additional parameters including the severity of **marrow fibrosis**, karyotype and **gene mutations**. Scoring systems have also been developed for the prediction of survival post-HSCT.

14.8 TREATMENT

Treatment of PMF entails both curative and symptomatic treatments. Allogeneic HSCT is the only curative treatment for eligible patients but is associated with significant transplant-related death, relapse and severe morbidity. Therefore, HSCT should only be considered for otherwise fit patients at high or very high risk of leukaemia transformation. For HSCT ineligible patients, symptomatic treatment targets anaemia, constitutional symptoms and splenomegaly.

Anaemia. Blood transfusion is the mainstay of treatment, and iron chelation should be considered in patients who need repeated transfusions. Androgens, prednisolone, danazol and thalidomide have been shown to improve anaemia in about 20% of patients, and the response is typically transient.

Constitutional symptoms. Constitutional symptoms are a major cause of morbidity in patients with advanced PMF. JAK inhibitors, including ruxolitinib and more recently, pacritinib, fedratinib and momelitinib, have been shown to be effective in relieving these symptoms and those associated with splenomegaly.

Splenomegaly. In the absence of anaemia or constitutional symptoms, hydroxyurea is the first-line treatment. JAK inhibitor ruxolitinib is also effective, but it is complicated by worsening anaemia and thrombocytopenia. In refractory patients, splenectomy or splenic irradiation should be considered.

14.9 KEY POINTS

1. Diagnosis of PMF includes clinicopathologic, cytogenetic and genetic parameters and exclusion of differential diagnoses.

2. Prognostic scores are available for the prediction of risk of leukaemia transformation and survival.
3. Allogeneic HSCT is the only curative treatment for eligible patients. Symptomatic treatment targets anaemia, constitutional symptoms and symptomatic splenomegaly.

ADDITIONAL READING

1. Tefferi A. Primary myelofibrosis: 2023 update on diagnosis, risk-stratification, and management. Am J Hematol 2023; 98: 801–821.

15 Myeloid Neoplasm with Germline Predisposition

15.1 CLINICAL SCENARIO

A 30-year-old woman presented with symptomatic anaemia for 2 months and was admitted to hospital for fever. She had episodes of limb purpura at age 16 years, and her platelet count was $100–140 \times 10^9/L$. However, she has declined bone marrow and follow up since then. Her elder sister has enjoyed good past health. However, their mother died of acute leukaemia, and her maternal grandmother also died of "blood cancer". One maternal uncle, who was in Germany, also died of blood cancer, one of his sons died of leukaemia at the age of 10 years and another son was recently diagnosed with leukaemia and has received haematopoietic stem cell transplantation (HSCT) in Germany (Figure 15.1).

15.2 INVESTIGATIONS AND PATIENT PROGRESS

Bone marrow aspiration showed acute myeloid leukaemia (AML) with maturation and normal cyto-genetics. Next generation sequencing (NGS) that focused on the myeloid panel showed mutations of *BCOR*, *BCORL1*, *EZH2* and *RUNX1*. In addition, there was deletion of exon 1 and 2 of *RUNX1*. Examination of the patient's buccal swab showed only deletion of exon 1 and 2 of *RUNX1* but not the other point mutations. The patient received induction chemotherapy and the "7+3" regimen and achieved complete remission. Subsequently, she received consolidation chemotherapy with high-dose cytarabine.

15.3 QUESTIONS

1. What is the problem?
2. What is the relevance of the patient's personal and family history?
3. How would the information affect the management?

15.4 PATIENT PROGRESS

The personal history of thrombocytopenia and family history of acute leukaemia on the maternal side strongly suggested germline predisposition with particular reference to *RUNX1* deletion. Exon 1 and 2 deletion of *RUNX1* was also detectable in the germline DNA of the patient's sister and the archival DNA sample of her mother. The overall picture was consistent with myeloid neoplasm with germline predisposition.

15.5 MYELOID NEOPLASM WITH GERMLINE PREDISPOSITION

Recent advances in genome sequencing have shed important light on our understanding of the germline predisposition of myelodysplastic syndrome (MDS) and AML, which are generally known to be acquired diseases. At present, three groups of inherited diseases have been character-ised that involve more than 10 specific gene mutations (Table 15.1).[1] Expectedly, the list of diseases will expand as the genetic basis of more patient cohorts is revealed. Recognising these disease

DOI: 10.1201/9781003325413-17

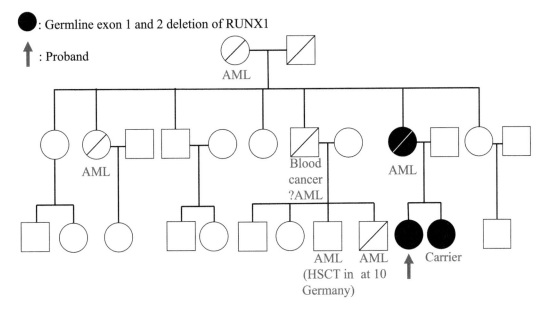

FIGURE 15.1 Pedigree of the myeloid malignancy with germline predisposition.

TABLE 15.1

Classification of Myeloid Neoplasms with Germline Predisposition

Without pre-existing platelet disorder or organ dysfunction

CEBPA

DDX41

TP53

With pre-existing platelet disorder

RUNX1

ANKRD26

ETV6

With potential organ dysfunction

GATA2

Bone marrow failure syndromes

Severe congenital neutropenia

Schwachman–Diamond syndrome

Fanconi Anaemia

Telomere Biology Disorders

RASopathies

Down syndrome

SAMD9

SAMD9L

Bi-allelic BLM

syndromes is clinically important as it facilitates accurate diagnosis for patients who present with platelet disorder or organ dysfunction and show a strong family history of MDS/AML. Moreover, genetic counselling can be offered to patients and their family members given the autosomal dominance in inheritance. Regular follow up and monitoring of asymptomatic carriers may be warranted because of their increased risk of developing MDS/AML. For patients with MDS/AML who are considered candidates for allogeneic HSCT, the inherited nature means that prospective donors from family should be screened to avoid transplantation of donor cells that carry the mutations, which may result in poor haematopoietic stem cell engraftment or function or donor cell leukaemia.

15.6   MYELOID NEOPLASMS WITH GERMLINE *RUNX1* MUTATION

Clinical presentation of patients with germline *RUNX1* mutation is variable. Typically, patients present with mild or moderate bleeding tendency in childhood with normal or mild thrombocytopenia. Most patients have impaired platelet aggregation towards collagen and epinephrine and a dense granule storage pool deficiency. Genetic anticipation has been reported. The nature of germline *RUNX1* mutations is highly variable, ranging from frameshift mutations and duplications to deletions and missense mutations. Progression to MDS/AML occurs at a median age of 33 years and may involve additional mutations. Haploinsufficiency of *RUNX1* arising from large deletions and acquisition of somatic mutation of the remaining *RUNX1* allele, as in this patient, appear to be common. Family members of patients with germline *RUNX1* mutation show variable penetrance of MDS/AML with a median of approximately 40%. Importantly, somatic *RUNX1* mutation is also a common occurrence in sporadic cases of MDS/AML. Careful evaluation of personal and family history of platelet disorders and MDS/AML is key to the distinction of myeloid neoplasms with germline predisposition.

15.7   KEY POINTS

1. Careful personal and detailed family history are important in the diagnosis of myeloid neoplasm with germline predisposition.
2. Accurate diagnosis is important for the management of patients and asymptomatic carriers, the decision on allogeneic HSCT and the choice of donors.
3. At least 10 gene mutations are associated with this group of diseases at present. Simultaneous evaluation of germline DNA from buccal swab or hair follicles from patients is essential.

ADDITIONAL READING

1. Peterson LC, Bloomfield CD, Niemeyer CM et al. Myeloid neoplasms with germline predisposition In: Swerdlow SH et al., eds. *WHO Classification of Tumours of Haematopoietic and Lymphoid Tissues.* International Agency for Research on Cancer 2017, pp. 122–128.

16 Langerhans Cell Histiocytosis

16.1 CLINICAL SCENARIO

A 45-year-old man with a history of asthma since childhood presented with a mass at the back of the neck, which had increased in size for 1 year. He was a non-smoker. Physical examination showed a soft and cystic lesion 6–7 cm in size. An incision biopsy showed deep dermis and subcutaneous tissue infiltrated by large histiocytes with reniform (kidney-shaped) and contorted nuclei and abundant cytoplasm. Many eosinophils were present in the background. The large histiocytes expressed diffuse reactivity to S100 protein, CD1a and CD207 (langerin), consistent with Langerhans cell histiocytosis (LCH) (Figure 16.1A).

Computed tomography (CT) showed multiple cystic lesions and nodules in both lungs (Figure 16.1B). There were also small roundish lytic lesions at the skull vault near midline. Magnetic resonance imaging (MRI) of the brain showed a 2-cm mass in the right temporal lobe. Lung biopsy showed emphysematous changes, with patchy fibrosis and the presence of some nodules of Langerhans cells. Cerebrospinal fluid was negative for malignant cells. The patient was treated with cytarabine with an initial pulmonary response, but shortly thereafter, there was disease progression in the liver and pelvic muscles as confirmed by liver and muscle biopsies. Subsequently, he received 5 courses of cladribine, resulting in complete disease resolution for at least 3 years at the time of writing.

16.2 QUESTIONS

1. What is the original cell of Langerhans cell histiocytosis?
2. What is the pathogenesis?
3. What is the treatment approach?

16.3 LANGERHANS CELL HISTIOCYTOSIS

Histiocytes refer to tissue-resident macrophages or dendritic cells that play pivotal roles in phagocytosis and antigen presentation. Langerhans cells (LCs) are tissue-resident macrophages of the skin that can take up apoptotic bodies and take on the role of dendritic cells and migrate to the lymph nodes where they present antigen to naïve T-cells.

Histologically, Langerhans Cell Histiocytosis (LCH) is characterised by the presence of clonal LCs with reniform nuclei that are positive for CD1a and CD207 admixed in an intense inflammatory infiltrate comprising macrophages, lymphocytes, eosinophils and multinucleated giant cells. These clonal LCs proliferate and infiltrate into virtually any organ system, with a predilection for skin, bones, lung, liver and brain. The cell of origin of LCH has remained elusive. Earlier studies showed that LCH might arise from neoplastic transformation of cutaneous LCs due to the presence of Birbeck granules in LCH cells that were once thought to be unique to epidermal LCs. More recently, *BRAF*V600E mutation has been identified in a small population of bone marrow haematopoietic progenitors from patients with LCH, and in mouse models, expression of *BRAF*V600E in haematopoietic progenitors generate LCH-like disease, suggesting that LCH might arise from haematopoietic precursors. Mutated haematopoietic progenitors and phagocytes undergo cellular changes and secrete cytokines, including the senescence-associated secretory phenotype (SASP), which results in LCH phenotypes in a cell autonomous and non-cell autonomous fashion (Figure 16.2A).

DOI: 10.1201/9781003325413-18

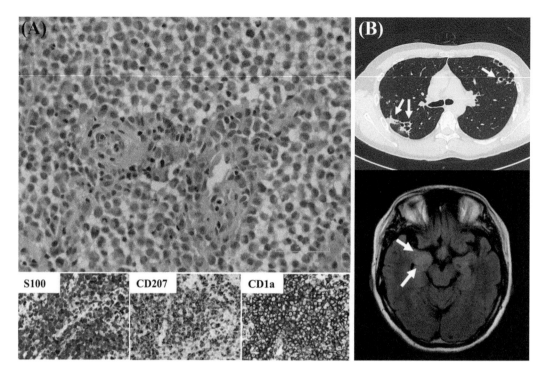

FIGURE 16.1 (A) H&E staining of the mass lesion in subcutaneous tissue showing dense infiltration by large histiocytes and increased eosinophils (upper panel). The histiocytes showed characteristic immunohistochemical features (lower panels). (B) Computed tomography of the thorax showing cystic lesions (arrows). Magnetic resonance imaging (MRI) showed a mass lesion (arrows) in the right temporal lobe. (*Figure 16.1A, courtesy of Dr. Rex Au Yeung.*)

Molecular pathogenesis. LCH is characterised by the activation of the MAP kinase pathway due to gain-of-function mutation of tyrosine kinases. Specifically, *BRAF*V600E occurs in about 60% of patients, and mutually exclusive mutations of upstream or downstream tyrosine kinases have also been identified (Figure 16.2B). Intriguingly, activation of the MAP kinase pathway is also evident even in patients without documented gene mutations.

Clinical presentation. The presentations of LCH are highly variable and depend on the sites of disease involvement. Lesions in the spleen, liver and bone marrow are associated with increased mortality and are considered high-risk sites. The extent of disease involvement can be categorised based on the number of lesions and organ systems, ranging from single lesions or single systems to multifocal lesions and multisystem involvement. **Cutaneous presentation** is most common and polymorphous, and patients may present with pruritus or ulcerative rash. **Skeletal involvement** may present with local pain or mechanical damage, classically with vertebra plana (complete collapse of vertebra). **Pulmonary presentation**, particularly among smokers, includes recurrent pneumothorax or obstructive pulmonary disease. **Hepatic involvement** may manifest as hepatomegaly or acute hepatitis and in chronic cases, sclerosing cholangitis. **Central nervous system (CNS) involvement** classically presents with sudden onset of diabetes insipidus due to a pituitary lesion, and those with more widespread CNS involvement may present with LCH-associated neurodegeneration.

Investigations. The initial investigation should focus on an accurate diagnosis of LCH based on an adequate tissue biopsy that shows not only the characteristic cellular features and immunophenotype of LCH cells but also the inflammatory backgrounds. Molecular diagnosis based on mutations of key tyrosine kinase of the MAP kinase pathway, particularly *BRAF*V600E, is helpful in confirming the diagnosis, although a negative mutation test does not rule out LCH. Subsequent

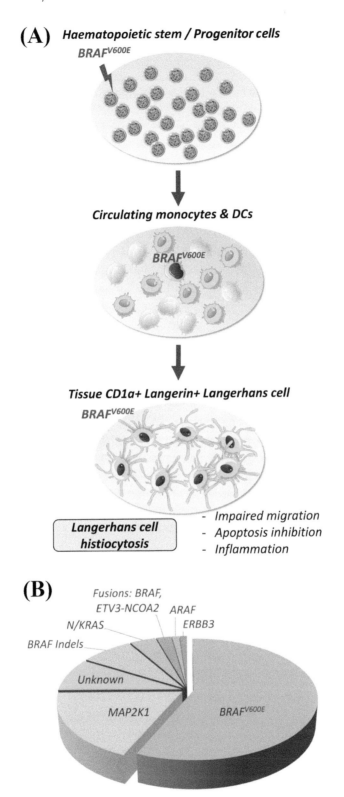

FIGURE 16.2 (A) Cell of origin in the Langerhans cell histiocytosis (LCH) pathogenesis. DC: Dendritic cell. (B) Mutation landscape of LCH.

diagnosis should focus on delineation of the extent of disease including a whole body Positron emission tomography/Computed tomography scan, high resolution CT scan of the thorax and brain MRI. Workup for endocrinopathy and diabetes insipidus is warranted.

Treatment. The treatment approach depends on the extent of disease. A solitary bone lesion is often treated with curettage, local steroid injection or irradiation, and a solitary cutaneous lesion can be irradiated or excised. Multifocal or multisystem diseases are managed by systemic treatment. A traditional regimen entails a protracted course (i.e., 12 months) of a combination of chemotherapy and corticosteroids. More recently, single agents such as cytarabine or purine analogues including cladribine or clofarabine have been used with success. As LCH is characterised by activating mutations of tyrosine kinase of the MAP kinase pathway, it also shows clinical responses to *BRAF*V600E and MEK inhibitors, especially for patients with relapsed or refractory diseases or those who are unfit for conventional chemotherapy.

16.4   OTHER HISTIOCYTOSIS

Histiocytoses comprise a diverse spectrum of rare diseases that share in common the activation of cellular signals, particularly the MAP kinase pathway and an increase in histiocytes. In addition to LCH, other examples include Erdheim–Chester Disease, Juvenile xanthogranuloma, Rosai–Dorfman disease and haemophagocytic lymphohistiocytosis. These diseases are distinct in their cell of origin, age of onset, predilection for organ involvement and, therefore, clinical presentation.

16.5   KEY POINTS

1. LCH is characterised histologically by the presence of clonal LCs with specific immunohistochemical features and inflammatory infiltrate.
2. Clinical presentations of LCH are variable, depending on the sites of involvement.
3. LCH is characterised by activating mutations of the MAP kinase pathway, including *BRAF*V600E, which provides a means of therapeutic targeting.

ADDITIONAL READINGS

1. Emile JF, Cohen-Aubart F, Collin M et al. Histocyotosis. Lancet 2021; 398: 157–170.
2. McClain KL, Bigenwald C, Collin M et al. Histiocytic disorders. Nat Rev Dis Primers 2021; 7(73): 1–26.

Lymphoid Malignancy

17 Diffuse Large B-Cell Lymphoma

17.1 CLINICAL SCENARIO

A 60-year-old man with good past health presented with a right neck mass 6 weeks ago. The mass showed progressive increase in size. There was no constitutional symptom. Physical examination showed an enlarged right cervical lymph node, which was non-tender and rubbery in consistency. His complete blood counts and baseline biochemistry, including lactate dehydrogenase (LDH), were within normal limits.

Positron emission tomography/computed tomography (PET/CT) scan showed an enlarged right submandibular lymph node, which measured $2 \times 2.3 \times 1.9$ cm in size with SUVmax of 31.17 (Figure 17.1A). Mild symmetrical fluorodeoxyglucose (FDG) uptakes were noted in the bilateral tonsils. There was no other metabolically active lesion.

The patient had a fine needle aspiration, which showed "atypical lymphoid proliferation" and subsequently underwent excisional biopsy. The enlarged lymph node was diffusely infiltrated by large atypical lymphoid cells resembling centroblasts and immunoblasts. They were positive for B-cell marker CD20, negative for CD10 but positive for MUM1. Most of these lymphoid cells were positive for C-MYC and BCL2 but negative for BCL6. A diagnosis of diffuse large B-cell lymphoma was made, supporting a non-germinal center B-cell-like (non-GCB) subtype with double expression of C-MYC and BCL2 (Figure 17.1B). His bone marrow was negative for lymphoma involvement. He was treated with R-CHOP × 6 courses (see the following) and achieved a complete remission thereafter.

17.2 DIFFUSE LARGE B-CELL LYMPHOMA—OVERVIEW

Diffuse large B-cell lymphoma (DLBCL) is the most common non-Hodgkin Lymphoma (NHL), accounting for one-third of cases. It is a heterogenous group of diseases with distinct clinicopathologic features that share in common the presence of medium or large abnormal lymphoid cells expressing **B-cell** marks (*viz.*, CD19, CD20, CD22, CD79a, PAX5 and surface and cytoplasmic immunoglobulins) whose nuclei are comparable to those of normal macrophages or are twice the size of those of a normal lymphocyte (**Large**) with a diffuse growth pattern in the enlarged lymph nodes (**Diffuse**). Distinct subtypes of lymphomas with the presence of neoplastic large B-cells have been recognised by, for instance, the peculiar sites of involvement (central nervous system [CNS], thymus, cutaneous site of leg, pleural effusion and vasculature), association with specific viral infection (Epstein–Barr virus [EBV] and human herpesvirus-8 [HHV-8]), molecular aberration (*IRF4* rearrangement and *ALK* expression), pathologic features (T-cell/histiocyte-rich and plasmablastic) and specific clinicopathologic features (associated with chronic inflammation and lymphomatoid granulomatosis). A distinct subset shows a high proliferative index and *MYC* and *BCL2* and/or *BCL6* gene rearrangement, known as high-grade B-cell lymphoma. The majority of cases that do not fall into these subtypes are collectively known as DLBCL-not otherwise specified (NOS).

17.3 AETIOLOGY

The aetiology of DLBCL-NOS is largely unknown. Most cases arise *de novo*, and others arise from underlying low-grade lymphoproliferative diseases including follicular lymphoma, marginal zone lymphoma or chronic lymphocytic leukaemia/small cell lymphoma. Immunocompromised patients are known to be at risk, and in these cases, EBV infection is frequently identified.

DOI: 10.1201/9781003325413-20

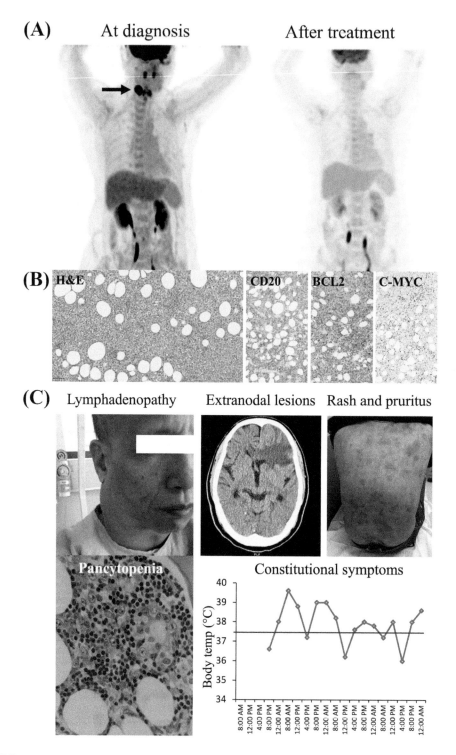

FIGURE 17.1 (A) Positron emission tomography/Computed tomography (PET/CT) scan of the patient before and after treatment. The initial site of disease is shown by an arrow. (B) Pathological features of the lymph node, which was replaced diffusely by large B-cell lymphoma cells expressing CD20 and BCL2 and some that also expressed C-MYC. (C) Diverse clinical presentations of diffuse large B-cell lymphoma. (*Figure 17.1B, courtesy of Dr. Rex Au Yeung.*)

17.4 CELL OF ORIGIN

DLBCL-NOS is classified by its cell of origin (COO) based on its distinct gene expression profile (GEP) pertinent to normal B-cell counterparts and comprises germinal centre B-cell-like (GCB) and activated B-cell-like (ABC). In general, the GCB type is more prevalent and showed significantly better clinical outcome in the pre-rituximab era. With the use of rituximab, the prognostic difference between GCB and ABC has become modest. As GEP is not widely accessible in clinical practice, COO is commonly defined by using immunohistochemistry (IHC) based upon expression of CD10, BCL6 and IRF4/MUM1 (Han's algorithm).

17.5 MOLECULAR LANDSCAPE

DLBCL-NOS has also been defined by its genetic signature that entails heavy immunoglobulin and light chain gene rearrangement, gene mutations, copy number variation and chromosomal translocations. Some of these features are associated with the specific COO. Lymphoma with *MYC, BCL2* and/or *BCL6* translocations (double or triple hit lymphoma) is now called high-grade B-cell lymphoma and is associated with an inferior outcome when treated with conventional immunochemotherapy R-CHOP. The prognostic importance and clinical applications of genetic signatures in DLBCL-NOS remain to be determined.

17.6 CLINICAL PRESENTATION

A majority of patients with DLBCL-NOS present with solitary or generalised lymphadenopathy that is characteristically non-tender and rubbery in consistency. Some patients may present with symptoms pertaining to extranodal involvement as space-occupying lesions or source of bleeding. Patients with bone marrow involvement may present with pancytopenia and/or constitutional symptoms (i.e., fever, night sweats and weight loss > 10% body weight in < 6 months) (Figure 17.1C).

17.7 MANAGEMENT

An accurate diagnosis of lymphoma requires sufficient tissues for histological evaluation, immunohistochemical staining, fluorescence in-situ hybridisation (FISH) and genetic analysis. In most circumstances, fine needle biopsy is not useful and often results in a delayed diagnosis. In patients in whom lymphoma is suspected, excisional biopsy of the enlarged lymph node is highly recommended whenever possible. Once a diagnosis is made, bone marrow examination and PET/CT scan are needed for lymphoma staging. The treatment paradigms for DLBCL-NOS demonstrate the wide array of modalities that are currently available in medical oncology. Rituximab, cyclophosphamide, hydroxydaunorubicin, oncovin and prednisolone (R-CHOP) has been the mainstay of treatment. For double hit or double expressor DLBCL, multi-agent chemotherapeutic regimens more intensive than R-CHOP are commonly used, but the optimal treatments have not been defined.

Patients who fail to respond to first-line treatment or who relapse after initial response are treated with salvage chemotherapy. Chemo-sensitive cases are treated with high-dose chemotherapy followed by autologous haematopoietic stem cell (HSC) rescue. Patients who do not respond well to these treatments or who relapse < 12 months after HSC rescue used to have an extremely poor prognosis. However, a number of new treatments are currently available that have shown to improve outcomes for patients with relapse/refractory DLBCL-NOS:

Immunomodulatory agent/Naked antibody: Tafasitamab against CD19 in combination with lenalidomide.

Antibody drug conjugate: Monoclonal antibody targeting lymphoma surface antigen conjugated with a payload that provides cytotoxic effect. Polatuzumab vedotin against CD79b conjugated with MMEA in combination with benadmustine and rituximab; Loncastuximab tesirine against CD19 conjugated with a pyrrolobenzodiazepine dimer toxin.

Exportin 1 inhibitor: Exportin 1 is a nuclear exporter that mediates the export of tumour-suppressor proteins, including p53, out of the nucleus. Exportin 1 inhibitor selinexor retains these suppressor proteins within the nucleus, restoring their tumour-suppressor function.

Bi-specific T-cell engagers: These antibodies bring effector T-cells (CD3) to lymphoma cells expressing CD20. In particular, glofitamab has been approved for the treatment of DLBCL, whereas mosunetuzumab has been approved for follicular lymphoma.

Chimeric antigen receptor-modified (CAR) T-cells: Axicabtagen ciloleucel (axi-cel) and tisagenlecleucel (tisa-cel) have been approved. Long-term remission is possible, and they appear to overcome adverse risk factors including unfavourable COO and the double expression of MYC and BCL2/BCL6. Limitations include the need for the successful apheresis of autologous T-cells, limited availability of a cellular therapy facility in treating institutes and high operative costs.

17.8   PROGNOSTICATION

Prognoses of DLBCL used to be defined on clinical grounds based on the International Prognostic Index (IPI), which entails the age (**A**) and performance (**P**) status of patients, their serum **LDH** level, the presence of extranodal (**E**) diseases and staging (**S**; acronym APLES). Currently, immunohistochemistry (IHC) that ascertains the COO and examines the protein expression of MYC, BCL2 and BCL6 has become standard laboratory practice in the evaluation of DLBCL-NOS. Specifically, the GCB subtype may be associated with better treatment response to R-CHOP, whereas MYC and BCL2 or BCL6 expression (double or triple expressor, distinct from chromosomal translocation, in which *MYC* and *BCL2* or *BCL6* translocation are known as double or triple hit lymphoma, respectively) are associated with inferior outcomes after R-CHOP.

17.9   KEY POINTS

1. DLBCL is the most common lymphoma type and is highly heterogeneous with different COOs and clinicopathologic and prognostic features.
2. Excisional biopsy is recommended whenever possible for accurate diagnosis and classification of lymphoma.
3. Treatments of DLBCL include monoclonal antibody, chemotherapy and cellular therapy. New treatments particularly for relapsed and refractory cases have emerged.

ADDITIONAL READINGS

1. Danilov AV, Magagnoli M, Matasar MJ. Translating the biology of diffuse large B-cell lymphoma into treatment. Oncologist 2022; 27: 57–66.
2. Gascoyne RD, Gampo E, Jaffe ES et al. Diffuse large B-cell lymphoma, NOS. In: Swerdlow SH et al., eds. *WHO Classification of Tumours of Haematopoietic and Lymphoid Tissues.* International Agency for Research on Cancer 2017, pp. 291–297.

18 Waldenström Macroglobulinaemia

18.1 CLINICAL SCENARIO

A 65-year-old housewife presented with low-grade fever ($< 38°C$) and malaise for two months. Her father died of carcinoma of the oesophagus. She carried the thalassaemia trait and had a history of osteoporosis, trigeminal neuralgia and benign thyroid nodules treated by hemithyroidectomy. Physical examination was unremarkable. Her baseline haemoglobin level was 10–11 g/dL.

18.2 LABORATORY REPORTS

	Results	Reference Range	Units
Haemoglobin	7.9	11.5–14.8	g/dL
White cell count	4.16	3.89–9.93	10^9/L
Platelet count	219	167–396	10^9/L
Immunoglobulin G	471	819–1725	mg/dL
Immunoglobulin A	49	70–386	mg/dL
Immunoglobulin M	4260	55–307	mg/dL
Paraprotein IgM/κ	2118	Absent	mg/dL

Bone marrow aspiration showed abnormal infiltration by small lymphocytes, lymphoplasmacytic lymphocytes and scattered plasma cells (Figure 18.1A). Flow cytometry demonstrated κ-restricted B-cells that were CD19+ and CD20+ but negative for CD5, CD10 and CD23. Molecular analysis showed positivity for *MYD88* p.L265P mutation. Positron emission tomography/Computed tomography (PET/CT) showed a few intra-abdominal lymph nodes with mild fluorodeoxyglucose (FDG) activity.

18.3 QUESTIONS

1. What is the likely diagnosis?
2. What is the risk to the patient?
3. What is the treatment approach?

18.4 CLINICAL PROGRESS

The patient was diagnosed Waldenström Macroglobulinaemia (WM). She was given a combination of rituximab and bendamustine, which she tolerated very well. There was a gradual decrease in immunoglobulin (Ig) M level (Figure 18.1B), and her fever subsided after the first course.

18.5 WALDENSTRÖM MACROGLOBULINAEMIA

WM is an indolent B-cell lymphoproliferative disease that arises from a post-germinal centre B-cell that has undergone somatic hypermutation and has acquired a lymphoplasmacytoid phenotype and IgM secretory capacity. The neoplastic cells retain expression of mature B-cell markers, such as CD20 and surface IgM, which are normally lost in normal plasma cells.

DOI: 10.1201/9781003325413-21

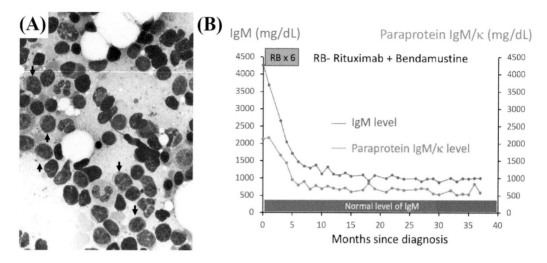

FIGURE 18.1   (A) Bone marrow infiltration by small lymphocytes, lymphoplasmacytic lymphocytes (arrows) and scattered plasma cells in Waldenström macroglobulinaemia (Wright-Giemsa × 1000). (B) The response of immunoglobulin (Ig) M and paraprotein IgM/κ to rituximab and bendamustine combination treatment.

18.6   CLINICAL MANIFESTATIONS

WM primarily affects the elderly with a median age of onset at 60–70 years. Many patients have preceding IgM monoclonal gammopathy of unknown significance (MGUS). Clinical presentations are non-specific. Patients can also be asymptomatic. The most common presentation is fatigue related to anaemia. Other patients may present with constitutional symptoms or symptoms related to the following conditions:

Peripheral neuropathy. This presents as a distal symmetric and slowly progressive senso-rimotor polyneuropathy characterised by paraesthesia and weakness. It is multi-factorial, including direct infiltration of nerves by monoclonal protein, malignant B-cells and amy-loidosis; IgM binds to myelin-associated glycoprotein (MAG) and cryoglobulinaemia.

Bing Neel syndrome. This is a rare manifestation that results from direct infiltration of the central nervous system by neoplastic lymphoid cells. Patients may present with headaches, cognitive or cranial nerve deficits, paresis, and psychiatric symptoms.

Cryoglobulinaemia. Cryoglobulins refer to immunoglobulins that precipitate at < 37°C and redissolve at higher temperatures. Cryoglobulinaemia is associated with diverse diseases including WM in which the temperature-sensitive insolubility, i.e., cryoglobulin activity, is caused by paraprotein IgM in a concentration-dependent manner. Many patients are asymptomatic, but some may present with weakness, purpura, arthralgias, Raynaud's phe-nomenon, acrocyanosis, ulcers, livedo reticularis and proliferative glomerulonephritis.

Bleeding tendency. Patients with WM may develop acquired Von Willebrand Disease. High serum viscosity increases the shear force that may alter the conformation of large Von Willebrand Factor multimers, thereby enhancing their susceptibility to cleavage by ADAMTS13. Amyloidosis associated with WM may lead to Factor X deficiency due to its adsorption to amyloid fibrils.

Hyperviscosity. Serum viscosity is normally 1.4 to 1.8 centipoise (cp), with water being 1 cp. Hyperviscosity syndrome may occur when serum viscosity is above 4 cp when serum IgM, which exists as pentamers, is at an extremely high concentration. Patients with hypervis-cosity may present with mucosal bleeding, especially involving the nose and gingiva; it may also include visual abnormalities due to central retinal vein occlusion and neurological abnormalities including somnolence, diplopia, dizziness, headache and hearing.

Haemolytic anaemia. Monoclonal IgM in WM can bind to the I or i antigen of red blood cells at lower-than-core body temperature, usually at extremities including fingers, toes, nose and ears, resulting in red cell agglutination (the antibody is known as cold agglutinin). Patients may present with acrocyanosis upon exposure to cold. IgM can also fix complement due to its pentameric structure, which results in autoimmune haemolytic anaemia. Patients may present with symptomatic anaemia and haemoglobinuria. Many patients present with cold agglutinin disease years before developing full-blown WM.

18.7 DIAGNOSIS

WM is defined as i) lymphoplasmacytic lymphoma (LPL) involving bone marrow (BM) and sometimes the lymph nodes and spleen and ii) is associated with a monoclonal IgM protein at any concentration. Pathologically, LPL entails a spectrum of B-cell differentiation in BM, including small lymphocytes, "plasmacytoid" lymphocytes and plasma cells. The relative predominance of these populations varies, but in total, they should account for more than 10% of nucleated cells. More than 90% of patients carry a gain-of-function *MYD88* L265P mutation, and about 30% of patients carry CXCR4 mutations that lead to truncated protein. The presence of gene mutation supports but does not define the diagnosis of WM as this may occur in other lymphoma subtypes.

18.7.1 MANAGEMENT OF WALDENSTRÖM MACROGLOBULINAEMIA

The management approach depends on the presence of symptoms and complications, the IgM level, patient tolerability and expected quality of life and the cost or reimbursement status of therapeutic agents. Asymptomatic patients can be closely monitored without treatment. Patients with symptomatic hyperviscosity and cryoglobulinaemia should receive plasma exchange for a rapid reduction of monoclonal IgM. As most patients are elderly, definitive treatment should aim at reducing IgM to a safe level, relieving symptoms and preventing complications rather than disease eradication.

Anti-CD20, e.g., rituximab, monotherapy is of limited efficacy, but its combination with chemotherapeutic agents can bring about a high response rate (> 70%) and long duration of progression-free survival that typically lasts for years. Treatment is given for 6 courses, and responses can be evaluated by the decrease in IgM, improvement in symptoms and complications, lymphadenopathy or hepatosplenomegaly. Bendamustine, a drug with both alkylating and antimetabolite activities, is commonly used. Combination chemotherapy, typically used for other lymphoma, e.g., cyclophosphamide, hydroxydaunorubicin (adriamycin), Oncovin (vincristine), prednisolone (CHOP) or its derivatives can also be considered but is associated with higher toxicity and less response durability.

More recently, novel therapeutic agents have been approved by the U.S. Food and Drug Administration (FDA) for the treatment of WM. Proteasome inhibitors, classically used for plasma cell dyscrasia, can be used in combination with rituximab with or without cyclophosphamide and/or dexamethasone. Bruton's tyrosine kinase inhibitor ibrutinib, classically used for chronic lymphocytic leukaemia, can also be employed as monotherapy or in combination with rituximab. These therapeutic agents have toxicity profiles different from chemotherapy, and their long-term efficacy remains to be determined.

18.8 KEY POINTS

1. WM is characterised by the presence of monoclonal IgM paraprotein, neoplastic B-cells of lymphoplasmacytoid phenotype in BM and *MYD88* L265P mutation in 90% of cases.
2. Clinical presentations of WM are diverse and non-specific, including anaemic and bleeding symptoms, cryoglobulinaemia and neurological deficits.

3. Treatment includes a combination of anti-CD20 monoclonal antibody and chemotherapy. Proteasome inhibitor and Bruton's tyrosine kinase inhibitor can also be used.

ADDITIONAL READINGS

1. Stone MJ, Pascual V. Pathophysiology of Waldenström's macroglobulinemia. Haematologica 2010; 95(3): 359–364.
2. Thomas SK. SOHO state of the art updates and next questions: Waldenström Macroglobulinemia—2021 update on management and future directions. Clin Lymphoma Myeloma Leuk 2022; 12(3): 1–9.
3. Castillo JJ, Treon SP. What is new in the treatment of Waldenstrom macroglobulinemia? Leukemia 2019; 33: 2555–2562.
4. Gertz MA. Waldenström macroglobulinemia: 2021 update on diagnosis, risk stratification, and management. Am J Hematol 2021; 96: 258–269.

19 Chronic Lymphocytic Leukaemia

19.1 CLINICAL SCENARIO

A 54-year-old businessman has had generalised lymphadenopathy since 2003 and has received chlorambucil from a private practitioner. He presented with worsening lymphadenopathy and night sweats for 6 months in 2017. Liver and spleen were not palpable.

19.2 LABORATORY REPORTS

	Results	Reference Range	Units
Haemoglobin	13.4	11.5–14.8	g/dL
White cell count	19.4	3.89–9.93	10^9/L
Neutrophil count	3.44	2.01–7.74	10^9/L
Lymphocyte count	15.2	1.06–3.61	10^9/L
Platelet count	139	167–396	10^9/L

Blood film showed numerous small, mature-looking lymphocytes with condensed chromatin and a high nuclear-cytoplasm (N/C) ratio. Smear cells were easily found (Figure 19.1A). Positron emission tomography/Computed tomography (PET/CT) scan showed enlarged lymph nodes about 3 cm in size in the neck, axillae and groin areas (Figure 19.1B).

19.3 QUESTIONS

1. What is the most likely diagnosis?
2. What is the management plan?
3. What complications may occur?

19.4 CLINICAL PROGRESS

Bone marrow examination was performed and showed a predominance of small lymphocytes with the characteristic immunophenotype of chronic lymphocytic leukaemia (CLL). Fluorescence in-situ hybridisation (FISH) analyses showed no evidence of chromosomal abnormalities associated with adverse (del[11q], trisomy 12, or del[17p]) or favourable (del[13q]) prognosis. The *immunoglobulin heavy-chain variable region* (*IGHV*) gene was mutated. The patient received 6 courses of immuno-chemotherapy (Fludarabine, Cyclophosphamide, Rituximab [FCR]) in 2017 that was complicated by pneumonia and an episode of cytomegalovirus (CMV) antigenaemia.

At the end of treatment, there was residual bone marrow lymphocytosis around 20% that had lost CD20 expression. There was no palpable lymphadenopathy or constitutional symptoms. PET/CT scan showed significant improvement in lymphadenopathy, which became eumetabolic with a size of up to 1 cm. There was no peripheral blood lymphocytosis. The patient has received treatment with Bruton's tyrosine kinase (BTK) inhibitor ibrutinib since then.

In 2023, he developed progressive lymphocytosis and a marked increase in lactate dehydrogenase (LDH) to 1200 IU/L (reference range: 150–300 IU/L). There was abnormally large lymphocyte

DOI: 10.1201/9781003325413-22

lymphocytosis. PET/CT scan showed enlarged and metabolically active para-aortic lymphadenopathy (Figure 19.1C). Bone marrow and CT-guided lymph node biopsy confirmed Richter transformation (Figures 19.1D and 19.1E). Next generation sequencing (NGS) showed two *TP53* mutations in his bone marrow.

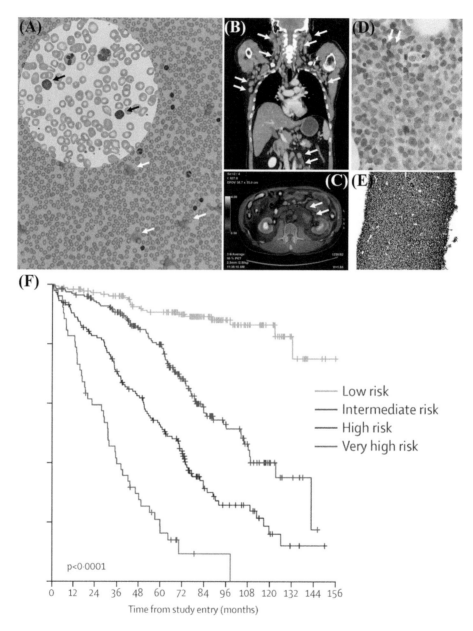

FIGURE 19.1 (A) Typical blood smear of chronic lymphocytic leukaemia (CLL) showing lymphocytosis (dark arrows) and smear cells (white arrows). (B) Positron emission tomography/Computed tomography (PET/CT) scan at presentation showing eumetabolic lymphadenopathy in the neck, axillae and groin regions. (C) PET/CT scan at Richter transformation showing metabolically active lymphadenopathy in the abdomen. (D) Bone marrow biopsy at transformation showing sheets of abnormal and large lymphoid cells. (E) These abnormal and large lymphoma cells expressing CD20. (F) Overall survival of the validation cohort in the CLL international prognostic index (CLL-IPI) model (from Ref 3 with permission): Low risk: 0–1; Intermediate risk: 2–3; High risk: 4–6; Very high risk: 7–10. (*Figure 1B and 1C, courtesy of Dr. Jamilla Li.*)

19.5 CHRONIC LYMPHOCYTIC LEUKAEMIA

CLL is the most common leukaemia in Caucasians with a median age of onset of 70 years[1] but is much less common in the Chinese. The ethnic difference is due to genetic predisposition as the disease prevalence is also low among Chinese immigrants in Western countries. Typically, patients present with lymphocytosis, lymphadenopathy, symptomatic anaemia or thrombocytopenia. CLL can be associated with autoimmune diseases including autoimmune haemolytic anaemia and immune thrombocytopenia.

19.6 DIAGNOSIS

A prerequisite for CLL diagnosis is the presence of lymphocytosis $> 5 \times 10^9/L$, with circulating clonal B-lymphocytes that persist for more than 3 months.[2] Morphologically, these lymphocytes are small and mature-looking. Smear or smudge cells, cell remnants lacking nuclei and cytoplasmic border are often present. Some patients present with a predominant nodal form known as small lymphocytic lymphoma (SLL) with the absence of or less than the defining level of clonal B-lymphocytosis for CLL. CLL and SLL should be considered diseases on the same spectrum with different presentations.

Subsequent investigations are needed to confirm the diagnosis and assess not only the stage and molecular characteristics of the disease but also organ function, co-morbidity and the premorbid functional state of patients that may guide treatment decisions. Diagnosis of CLL is confirmed by the typical immunophenotypes of CLL cells based on flow cytometry: CD5 (positive), CD23 (positive), FMC7 (negative), CD79b/CD22 (negative/weak) and surface immunoglobulin (negative/weak). Bone marrow examination is not essential, except for uncertain diagnosis or unexplained cytopenia. PET/CT scan at presentation is warranted to ascertain the extent of nodal involvement.

19.7 PROGNOSTICATION

Staging is mainly clinical and is defined by the Rai and the Binet systems (Tables 19.1 and 19.2, respectively). In both systems, late-stage disease is characterised by the presence of cytopenia, which reflects heavy tumour burden in the bone marrow. Cytogenetic changes are mostly defined by FISH. Specifically, deletions of chromosome 17p and 11q23 are associated with an inferior outcome. Trisomy 12 is associated with an intermediate outcome and deletion of chromosome 13q14 confers a superior long-term outcome. Mutations of *TP53* or *NOTCH1* are associated with inferior outcomes, whereas mutations of the *variable region of immunoglobulin gene heavy chain (IGHV)* confer favourable prognosis. A prognostic model incorporating patient factors, disease burden and molecular genetics, known as the CLL international prognostic index (CLL-IPI), has been developed (Table 19.3, Figure 19.1F).[3] (Courtesy of Dr. Thomas S.Y. Chan.) Transformation of CLL into aggressive lymphoma, known as Richter transformation, occurs in 2–9% of patients at a median of

---

TABLE 19.1

Rai Staging System

Stage	Clinical assessment
0	Asymptomatic lymphocytosis
I	Lymphocytosis with lymphadenopathy
II	Lymphocytosis with spleen and/or liver enlargement
III	Lymphocytosis with anaemia (haemoglobin $< 11 g/dL$)
IV	Lymphocytosis with thrombocytopenia (platelets $< 100 \times 10^9/L$)

TABLE 19.2
Binet Staging System

Stage	Clinical assessment
A	Lymphocytosis with < 3 groups of lymph node enlargement
B	Lymphocytosis with ≥ 3 groups of lymph node enlargement
C	Lymphocytosis with anaemia (haemoglobin < 10g/dL) and/or thrombocytopenia (platelets < 100×10^9/L)

TABLE 19.3
CLL IPI Scoring System

Variable	Adverse factor	Grading
Age	> 65 years	1
Clinical stage	Binet B/C or Rai I-IV	1
Del(17p) and/or *TP53* mutation	Deleted and/or mutated	4
IGHV mutation status	Unmutated	2
B2M level	> 3.5 mg/L	2

2–5 years after diagnosis. This is associated with an increase in the size and proliferation of CLL cells, progressively enlarged lymph nodes, raised LDH and the occurrence of constitutional symptoms. The median survival of patients with Richter transformation is measured in months. Rarely, CLL can be transformed into B-cell prolymphocytic leukaemia.

19.8 PRINCIPLE OF MANAGEMENT

Given the indolent nature of the disease and the advanced age of most patients, not all patients require immediate treatment. Indications for treatment in CLL include a rapid increase in lymphocyte count, bulky or obstructive lymphadenopathy, constitutional symptoms or cytopenia due to marrow infiltration by disease. Autoimmune haemolytic anaemia and immune thrombocytopenia, which are frequently associated with CLL, should be treated as such and are not indications for formal CLL treatment. Patients who are asymptomatic and without these indications can be managed conservatively by a watchful waiting approach.

Treatment modalities for CLL have changed substantially in recent years. The treatment goal is towards disease control, and cure is rarely achieved. In young and fit patients, immunochemotherapy used to be the standard of care (e.g., FCR) but has been largely replaced by less toxic and more specific targeted therapies including BTK inhibitor or a combination of BCL2 inhibitor venetoclax with anti-CD20 monoclonal antibody obinutuzumab. In relapsed or refractory cases, phosphoinositide 3-kinase (PI3k) inhibitor in combination with anti-CD20 monoclonal antibody can be used. In old and frail patients, obinutuzumab in combination with chlorambucil is tolerable and may be considered for disease control.

19.9 KEY POINTS

1. CLL patients typically present with lymphocytosis and lymphadenopathy. Anaemia and thrombocytopenia may occur due to autoimmunity or marrow infiltration.

2. Indications for CLL treatment include a rapid increase in lymphocyte count, bulky or obstructive lymphadenopathy, constitutional symptoms or cytopenia due to marrow infiltration by disease.
3. Prognosis of CLL is informed by disease staging, cytogenetics and genetics.
4. Bruton's tyrosine kinase inhibitor and a combination of anti-CD20 antibody and venetoclax are the mainstays of treatment.

ADDITIONAL READINGS

1. Cancer Stat Facts. *Leukemia—Chronic Lymphocytic Leukemia (CLL)*. National Cancer Institute. Surveillance Epidemiology and End Results Program (SEER). https://seer.cancer.gov/statfacts/html/clyl.html. Accessed on 2022 Sept 28.
2. Hallek M, Cheson BD, Catovsky D et al. iwCLL guidelines for diagnosis, indications for treatment, response assessment, and supportive management of CLL. Blood 2018; 131(25): 2745–2760.
3. The International CLL-IPI working group. An international prognostic index for patients with chronic lymphocytic leukaemia (CLL-IPI): a meta-analysis of individual patient data. Lancet Oncol 2016; 17: 779–790.

20 Hairy Cell Leukaemia

20.1 CLINICAL SCENARIO

A 58-year-old man with a history of renal stone was admitted for an episode of chest discomfort in March 2017. Three of his eldest sisters had carcinoma of the breast, ovary and colon. His paternal aunt died of leukaemia at age 70 years. Physical examination showed a palpable spleen tip.

20.2 LABORATORY REPORTS

	Results	References	Units
Haemoglobin	5.0	11.5–14.8	g/dL
White cell count	12.39	3.89–9.93	10^9/L
Platelet count	41	167–396	10^9/L
Neutrophil count	1.12	2.01–7.74	10^9/L
Monocyte count	0.01	0.18–0.65	10^9/L
Lymphocyte count	3.0	1.06–3.61	10^9/L
Abnormal lymphoid cells*	8.05	Absent	10^9/L

* Abnormal lymphoid cells were small to medium in size, with a moderate to high nuclear-to-cytoplasmic ratio, roundish nuclei, occasional inconspicuous nucleoli and pale cytoplasm with hairy cytoplasmic projections (Figure 20.1A).

Liver and renal function tests and lactate dehydrogenase were within normal limits.

20.3 QUESTIONS

1. What are the next investigations?
2. What is the likely diagnosis?
3. What is the management plan?

20.4 CLINICAL PROGRESS

Flow cytometry of the peripheral blood showed that the abnormal lymphoid cells were clonal B-cells that expressed CD19, CD20 (strong), CD22 and FMC7 and showed kappa light chain restriction. Bone marrow aspiration was unsuccessful, and trephine biopsy showed heavy infiltration by small to medium-sized abnormal lymphoid cells that were widely spaced with oval or indented nuclei (Figure 20.1B). Reticulin fibres were diffusely coarsened. Polymerase chain reaction (PCR) detected the presence of *BRAF* p.V600E mutation. A diagnosis of hairy cell leukaemia was made. Positron emission tomography/Computed tomography (PET/CT) scan showed splenomegaly (15.8 cm) with uniformly increased metabolic activity (SUVmax 3.3). Marrow uptake was also diffusely hypermetabolic (SUVmax 3.2–3.7) (Figure 20.1C).

The patient was treated with cladribine in March 2017, and repeated bone marrow examinations showed no abnormal infiltrate. His blood counts also improved. In 2023, he was found to have disease relapse with recurrent monocytopenia, abnormal circulating lymphocytes and splenomegaly. He was treated with cladribine again in June 2023 with a satisfactory response.

DOI: 10.1201/9781003325413-23

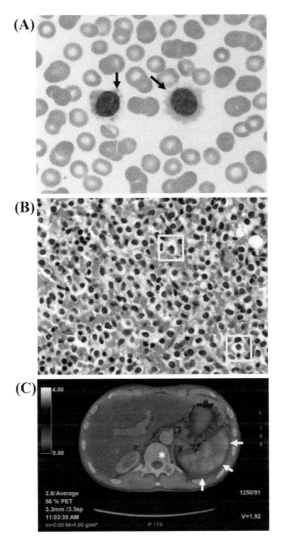

FIGURE 20.1 (A) Hairy cells in the peripheral blood showing cytoplasmic projections (arrows) (Wright-Giemsa × 1000). (B) Trephine biopsy histology of hairy cell leukaemia (H&E × 600) showing typical lymphoma cells with abundant cytoplasm and prominent cell borders, described as a fried-egg appearance (yellow squares). (C) Positron emission tomography/Computed tomography (PET/CT) scan of the patient showing splenomegaly (arrows) and bone marrow (asterisk) with increased metabolic activities.

20.5 HAIRY CELL LEUKAEMIA

Hairy cell leukaemia (HCL) is a rare but pathologically distinct lymphoid leukaemia characterised by pathognomonic circulating lymphoid cells with cytoplasmic (hairy) projections, characteristic bone marrow features, splenomegaly and *BRAF* V600E mutation of leukaemic cells.

Pathological characteristics. HCL is thought to be caused by *BRAF* V600E mutation of activated memory B-cells. The pathognomonic hairy cells are small to medium-sized lymphoid cells with an oval or indented nucleus. The characteristic cytoplasmic projections are circumferential in distribution, in contrast to the bipolar distribution in splenic marginal zone lymphoma (splenic lymphoma with villous lymphocytes). Bone marrow infiltration is characterised by widely spaced lymphoid cells with an increase in reticulin fibres, leading to "dry tap" in typical aspiration. The abnormal lymphoid cells are indicated by a distinct immunophenotypic profile. Mutation of *BRAF*V600E occurs in nearly all cases of HCL, which becomes an important diagnostic tool. The abnormal lymphoid cells are typically tartrate-resistant acid phosphatase (TRAP)-positive, but because of the availability of immunophenotype and genetic analyses, cytochemistry has become less important in the diagnostic algorithm.

Clinical characteristics. HCL is a disease of the middle-aged or elderly with a male preponderance. Most patients present with symptomatic anaemia, thrombocytopenia, fever and splenomegaly. Monocytopenia is characteristic and may contribute to the septic complications often seen in HCL.

Treatment. Purine analogues including cladribine and pentostatin are the mainstays of treatment, resulting in complete remission in most cases. Alternatively, interferon alpha has also been used. However, relapses are common, occurring in nearly 50% of cases. Late relapse as in this patient can be salvaged with the same treatment that brought about remission at diagnosis. In refractory cases, anti-CD20 monoclonal antibody, chemotherapy or BRAF inhibitors have been used as salvage.

20.6   HCL VARIANT

HCL variant (HCLv) encompasses B-cell lymphoproliferative diseases that share in common with HCL the villous projection of circulating lymphoid cells and the clinical features of splenomegaly, anaemia and thrombocytopenia. Unlike HCL, the abnormal lymphoid cells show a blastic or convoluted nucleus with prominent nucleoli, which are unusual in HCL. Moreover, there is a lack of monocytopenia, marrow fibrosis and *BRAF*V600E mutation. TRAP is negative, and purine analogues are usually ineffective in HCLv.

20.7   KEY POINTS

1. HCL is characterised by abnormal circulating lymphoid cells with villous projections, splenomegaly, monocytopenia, characteristic bone marrow features and *BRAF*V600E mutations.
2. Purine analogue cladribine is effective in inducing complete remission, but relapse is common.
3. Differential diagnoses of abnormal lymphoid cells with villous projections include splenic marginal zone lymphoma and HCL variants.

ADDITIONAL READING

1. Foucar K, Falini B, Stein H. Hairy cell leukaemia. In: Swerdlow SH et al., eds. *WHO Classification of Tumours of Haematopoietic and Lymphoid Tissues.* International Agency for Research on Cancer 2017, pp. 226–228.

21 Philadelphia Chromosome–Positive Acute Lymphoblastic Leukaemia

21.1 CLINICAL SCENARIO

A 60-year-old woman with good past health presented with a 1-week history of bone pain and fever.

21.2 LABORATORY REPORTS

	Results	References	Units
Haemoglobin	13.5	13.3–17.1	g/dL
White cell count	8.54	3.89–9.93	10^9/L
Platelet count	55	154–371	10^9/L
Lactate dehydrogenase	1182	128–245	IU/L

Liver and renal function tests: Unremarkable.
Blood films: Leukoerythroblastic blood picture. Blasts accounted for 7% of all white cells (Figure 21.1A, left upper panel).

Bone marrow showed markedly hypercellular marrow with blasts predominating at 95%. Flow cytometry showed that the blasts express CD34, Terminal deoxynucleotidyl transferase (Tdt) and B-lymphoid associated markers. They are largely negative for myeloid or T-lymphoid associated antigens.

21.3 QUESTIONS

1. What is the diagnosis?
2. What further investigations are needed?
3. What is the management plan?

21.4 PATIENT PROGRESS

A diagnosis of precursor B-cell acute lymphoblastic leukaemia (ALL) was made. Bone marrow (BM) cytogenetics and fluorescence in-situ hybridisation (FISH) showed the presence of t(9;22) (q34;q11.2). Reverse transcription polymerase chain reaction (RT-PCR) was positive for minor *BCR::ABL1* (e1a2) fusion transcript (Figure 21.1A, left lower, right upper and right lower panel). A formal diagnosis of Philadelphia chromosome–positive precursor B-cell ALL was confirmed. The patient was treated by a combination of tyrosine kinase inhibitor ponatinib and a multi-agent chemotherapy regimen HyperCVAD. BM examination 28 days after commencement of chemo-therapy showed morphologic complete remission (CR1). Her minimal (measurable) residual disease (MRD) by flow cytometry showed gradual decrease and became undetectable after 5 cycles (Figure 21.1B).

DOI: 10.1201/9781003325413-24

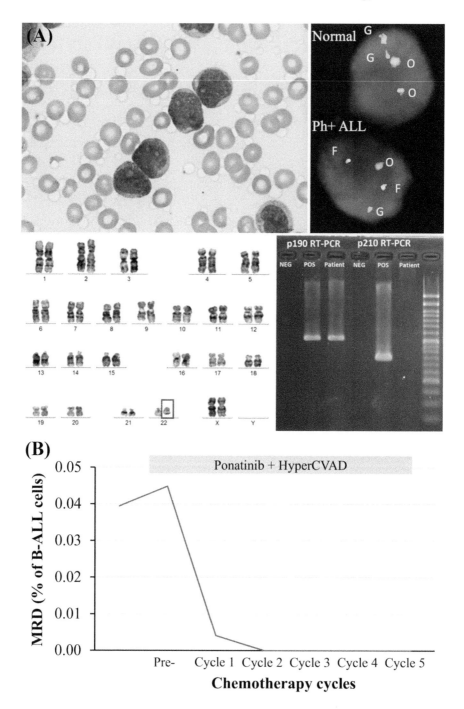

FIGURE 21.1 (A) (Left upper) Blood smear showing the presence of blast cells in Philadelphia chromosome–positive acute lymphoblastic leukaemia (Ph+ ALL) (Wright-Giemsa × 1000); (Left lower) Cytogenetic study showing the presence of t(9;22) translocation in this female patient, resulting in the formation of Philadelphia chromosome (red rectangle); (Right upper) Interphase fluorescence in-situ hybridisation (FISH) by BCR::ABL1 Dual Colour Dual Fusion probe showing a positive 1G1O2F signal pattern in the lower cell and normal 2G2O signal pattern in the upper cell. Key: Green (G) probe targets *BCR* gene locus at the 22q11.2 region, orange (O) probe targets *ABL1* gene locus at the 9q34 region and the green orange fusion (F) signal is yellow. (Right lower) Reverse transcription polymerase chain reaction (RT-PCR) showing positive detection of e1a2 p190 fusion transcript but negative for p210 fusion transcript. Pos: Positive; Neg: Negative. (B) Minimal (measurable) residual disease (MRD) response to a combination of ponatinib and chemotherapy hyperCVAD in this patient.

21.5   PRECURSOR B-CELL ALL

Precursor B-cell ALL arises from neoplastic transformation of a precursor lymphoid cell committed to B-cell lineage. It occurs primarily in children and is associated with good prognosis. In adults, precursor B-cell ALL is associated with less favourable outcomes. Most patients present with BM disease, bone pain and marrow failure. Involvement of lymph nodes and hepatosplenomegaly is frequent. Unlike precursor T-cell ALL, involvement of mediastinum is uncommon. Diagnosis depends on the presence of lymphoblasts in blood and BM, and immunophenotyping of lymphoblasts is essential to ascertain their origin from precursor B-cells. The degree of differentiation of lymphoblasts varies from early (pro-B-cells) and intermediate (common B-ALL) to late stage (pre-B ALL). Tdt, which is involved in T-cell receptor (TCR) and immunoglobulin heavy chain (IgH) rearrangement, is characteristically expressed in ALL but not in mature lymphoid neoplasms or acute myeloid leukaemia. Cytogenetics or FISH analysis is essential to identify recurrent genetic abnormalities underlying precursor B-cell ALL.

21.6   PHILADELPHIA CHROMOSOME–POSITIVE ALL

Philadelphia chromosome (Ph) is identified in up to 30% of adult patients with precursor B-cell ALL but is rare in childhood cases. It arises from a balanced translocation between chromosome 9 and chromosome 22, leading to the fusion between *BCR* on chromosome 22 and *ABL1* on chromosome 9. The fusion gene *BCR::ABL1* encodes for a constitutively activated tyrosine kinase, which is the driver of leukaemogenesis. Three variants of the *BCR::ABL1* genes have been described, namely, p190, p210 and p230, with the numbers indicating their respective molecular weight in kDa. In Ph+ ALL, the p190 variant is the most common, and the p210 variant occurs in 20% to 30% of cases. This contrasts with chronic myeloid leukaemia (CML) in which p210 is the predominant form.

21.7   TREATMENT OF PH+ ALL

Before the era of tyrosine kinase inhibitor (TKI), Ph+ ALL showed very poor prognosis upon treatment with conventional chemotherapy. Despite a high rate of initial remission, most patients subsequently relapse, and allogeneic haematopoietic stem cell transplantation (HSCT) is the only curative treatment. Prognosis of old and frail patients who are ineligible for standard treatment is dismal.

The advent of TKI, which was first developed for the treatment of CML, has provided treatment options and substantially improved the outcome of patients with Ph+ ALL. In young and fit patients, a combination of TKI with conventional chemotherapy is the mainstay of treatment and detection of MRD, based on flow cytometry or quantitative RT-PCR, and has become an important treatment endpoint. As ALL shows a propensity of central nervous system (CNS) involvement, CNS prophylaxis plays an integral part in most ALL regimens. Third-generation TKI ponatinib in this context appears to confer benefit on patients compared with first- or second-generation TKI, due to its higher efficacy and CNS penetration, and individuals who achieve negative MRD may have an equal or superior outcome to those who received consolidative allogeneic HSCT. Patients who fail to achieve negative MRD have the option of bi-specific T-cell engager blinatumomab, which brings CD3+ T-cells to the proximity of CD19 leukaemic precursor B-cells, and allogeneic HSCT should be considered. With this approach, long-term survival could be accomplished in a majority of patients. In old and frail patients ineligible for conventional treatment, TKI in combination with corticosteroid, low-intensity chemotherapy or blinatumomab is a reasonable option. Durable remission may be possible, but whether this approach is curative is currently unclear.

21.8   KEY POINTS

1. Philadelphia chromosome-positive ALL occurs in about 30% of adult cases with precursor B-cell ALL.
2. A combination of TKI with intensive chemotherapy (for young and fit patients) or with steroid or monoclonal antibody (for elderly patients) is the mainstay of treatment. Curability is possible without HSCT in the era of TKI.
3. MRD monitoring is essential for guiding treatment and the HSCT decision.

ADDITIONAL READINGS

1. Borowitz MJ, Chan JK, Downing JR et al. B-lymphoblastic leukaemia/lymphoma, not otherwise specified (NOS). In: Swerdlow SH et al., eds. *WHO Classification of Tumours of Haematopoietic and Lymphoid Tissues.* International Agency for Research on Cancer 2017, pp. 200–202.
2. Wieduwilt MJ. Ph+ ALL in 2022: is there an optimal approach? Hematology Am Soc Hematol Educ Program 2022 Dec 9; 2022(1): 206–212.

22 Natural Killer Cell Lymphoma

22.1 CLINICAL SCENARIO

A 47-year-old housewife with good past health presented with nasal blockade, occasional epistaxis and runny nose for two years. She consulted an ENT surgeon, and nasal endoscopy showed extensive granulation over the lateral nasal cavity involving the entire left nasal cavity and right anterior septum. Physical examination showed matted lymph nodes in the left cervical region. Biopsy of the left nasal cavity showed abnormal natural killer (NK) cells positive for CD3ε, CD56, TIA-1 and EBER, characteristic of NK/T-cell lymphoma, nasal type (Figures 22.1A–22.1F). Biopsy of the left cervical lymph node showed similar histology. Bone marrow showed the presence of histiocytes and haemophagocytosis without abnormal cellular infiltration. Positron emission tomography/Computed tomography (PET/CT) scan showed a hypermetabolic soft tissue mass filling the nasal cavity and lymph node in the left cervical region (Figure 22.1G). Plasma Epstein–Barr virus (EBV) DNA was 5.8 x 10^5 copies/mL.

22.2 QUESTIONS

1. What is extranodal NK/T-cell lymphoma?
2. What is the principle of management?
3. What is the prognosis?

22.3 CLINICAL PROGRESS

The patient received a combination of chemotherapy containing steroids and methotrexate, ifosfamide, L-asparaginase, etoposide, the SMILE protocol, and local radiotherapy (RT) and achieved complete remission based on her symptoms and interim PET/CT scan (Figure 22.1G). The plasma EBV DNA level became undetectable.

22.4 NK/T-CELL LYMPHOMA

NK/T-cell lymphoma arises from the neoplastic transformation of predominantly natural killer cells and rarely cytotoxic T-cells and is characterised by distinct morphological and immunophenotypic features. Characteristically, the lymphoma cells express CD56, a marker of NK cells, cytotoxic marker TIA-1 and cytoplasmic CD3. EBV infection is always present, which is suggestive of its pathogenetic significance, and has become a prerequisite for diagnosis. NK/T-cell lymphomas occur mainly in Asian and South American populations. Unlike other lymphoma types, the sites of involvement are predominantly extra-nodal. Various cytogenetic and genetic aberrations have been described, but none of them is pathognomonic of the diseases.

22.5 CLINICAL SUBTYPES OF NK/T-CELL LYMPHOMA

Three distinct categories are identified. About 80% of patients present with localised disease in the nose and upper aerodigestive tract, usually with minimal dissemination. This lymphoma is known as the **nasal type**. Patients may present with nasal obstruction and bleeding or destructive lesions in midline, hence the old name of lethal midline granuloma. A combination of L-asparaginase containing chemotherapeutic regimen and regional radiotherapy results in a favourable outcome. Overall, 15% of patients present with disseminated disease involving the skin, gastrointestinal tract

DOI: 10.1201/9781003325413-25

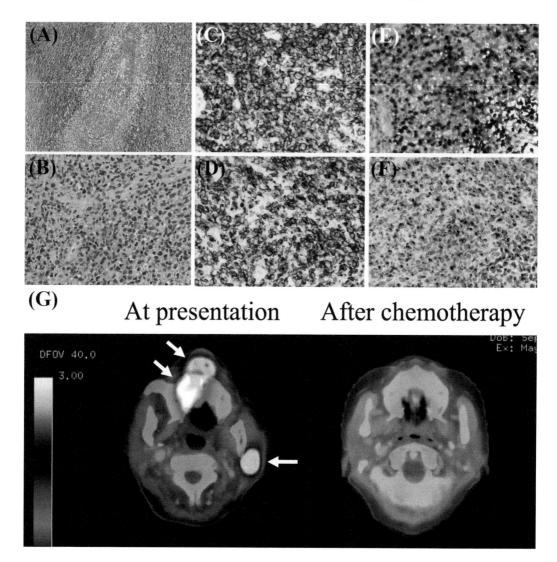

FIGURE 22.1 (A) Low power view of nasal biopsy showing invasion of a blood vessel by lymphoma cells. (B) High-power view of nasal biopsy showing invasion by abnormal NK cells, which were characterised as (C) CD56 positive, (D) Cytoplasmic CD3ε positive, (E) EBER positive and (F) Cytotoxic marker TIA positive. (G) PET/CT scan showing the response to combination chemo-irradiation. (*Figures 22.1A–22.1F, courtesy of Dr. Rex Au Yeung.*)

and testes, and this lymphoma is known as the **non-nasal type**. Constitutional symptoms are often present. Relapse after chemotherapy is frequently seen, and eligible patients may benefit from allogeneic haematopoietic stem cell transplantation at first complete remission. In total, 5% of patients present primarily with aggressive bone marrow disease and hepatosplenomegaly. This is known as **aggressive NK cell leukaemia**. Patients are notoriously refractory to conventional chemotherapy, and they often succumb to the disease within weeks. In all three subtypes, bone marrow haemophagocytosis may be present.

22.6   KEY POINTS

1. NK/T-cell lymphoma shows a significantly higher incidence in Asia and South America.
2. Epstein–Barr Virus infection is always present.
3. There are three distinct clinical subtypes: Nasal, non-nasal NK cell lymphoma and aggressive NK cell leukaemia.

ADDITIONAL READING

1. Chan JKC, Quintanilla-Martinez L, Ferry JA. Extranodal NK/T-cell lymphoma, nasal type. In: Swerdlow SH et al., eds. *WHO Classification of Tumours of Haematopoietic and Lymphoid Tissues.* International Agency for Research on Cancer 2017, pp. 368–371.

23 Mycosis Fungoides

23.1 CLINICAL SCENARIO

A 32-year-woman with good past health presented with erythematous rash in the buttocks and back of thighs since January 2019. Skin biopsy showed dense infiltration by small to large lymphocytes, which were predominantly CD3+ and CD4+ cells. CD30 expression varied from weak to moderate staining. The diagnosis was folliculotropic mycosis fungoides (MF) (Figure 23.1A). Bone marrow (BM) showed no lymphoma involvement, and Positron emission tomography/Computed tomography scan showed only metabolic activity over the incision site. She received phototherapy and topical steroid between March and July 2019 with initial response that subsequently fluctuated, and she was given repeated sessions of phototherapies.

The patient complained of worsening rash on the back and a new facial rash in June 2021. Repeated skin biopsy of the face and back showed the presence of sheets of large atypical lymphoid cells consistent with MF in large cell transformation. Flow cytometry of peripheral blood showed no abnormal lymphoid cells. A repeat PET/CT scan showed multifocal hypermetabolic dermal thickening in the face, trunk and lower limbs (Figure 23.1B, left panels). There were shotty and bilateral lymph nodes at the axillae and inguinal regions. Physical examination showed no palpable lymph nodes or organomegaly. The patient was treated with anti-CD30 monoclonal antibody with rapid improvement of the skin lesions after the first dose, and she continued treatment up to 16 cycles (Figure 23.1B, right panels).

23.2 QUESTIONS

1. What is mycosis fungoides?
2. What is the prognosis?
3. What is the treatment approach?

23.3 MYCOSIS FUNGOIDES

Unlike Hodgkin lymphoma that shows predilection for lymph node involvement, non-Hodgkin lymphoma (NHL) is more variable in its involvement. A rare form of NHL affects primarily the skin, also known as cutaneous T-cell lymphoma (CTCL), of which MF is the most common subtype and represents 50% of cases. In the presence of extensive skin involvement and circulating clonal T-cells with characteristic cerebriform nuclei, also known as Sézary cells, the condition is known as Sézary syndrome. Sézary syndrome occurs in about 5% of CTCL.

23.4 CLINICAL PRESENTATION

MF is an indolent CD4+ CTCL characterised by well-demarcated and pruritic cutaneous patches or plagues that in some patients, progress to mushroom-like tumours, hence the misnomer mycosis fungoides ("mushroom-like fungal disease"). In the later stage, patients may develop lymphadenopathy and hepatosplenomegaly.

23.5 STAGING OF MYCOSIS FUNGOIDES

Although the staging of classical Hodgkin lymphoma (cHL) and most NHL is based on the Ann Arbor System, the staging of MF is based on the TNMB system, which takes into consideration,

                                                   DOI: 10.1201/9781003325413-26

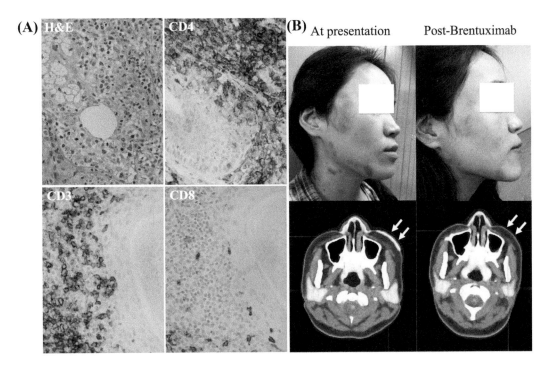

FIGURE 23.1 (A) Histological features of mycosis fungoides showing infiltration by small to large lymphocytes, which were predominantly CD3+ and CD4+. (B) Photographs of the patient (upper panels) and Positron emission tomography/Computed tomography (PET/CT) (lower panels) before and after treatment with anti-CD30 monoclonal antibody are shown. (*Figure 23.1A, courtesy of Dr.Rex Au Yeung.*)

on aggregate, skin (T) (T, surface area involved and cutaneous tumours), lymph nodes (N, reactive or lymphoma involved) and visceral (M) and blood (B, percentage of circulating lymphoma cells) involvement. The overall stage of MF ranges from early (IA-IIA) to advanced (IIB-IVB) stages.

Prognosis. A number of factors are of prognostic significance. At the advanced stage, histological features of large cell transformation and folliculotropic subtypes and raised serum lactate dehydrogenase (LDH) at presentation are associated with inferior prognosis.

Investigations. Investigations are for diagnostic and prognostic purposes and entail histologic, laboratory (LDH), imaging and molecular tests. Skin biopsy is essential to confirm the diagnosis. Pathognomonic features of cutaneous lesions include Paultrier microabscess, which refers to the intra-epidermal collection of abnormal lymphocytes. Molecular tests to identify T-cell receptor (TCR) rearrangement are needed to ascertain clonality. Excisional biopsy should be performed for palpable lymph nodes to distinguish between dermatopathic (reactive) changes versus lymphoma involvement. Examination of peripheral blood smear and flow cytometry is used to detect circulating lymphoma cells with characteristic cerebriform nuclei and immunophenotype. A raised LDH is of prognostic significance. PET/CT is needed to evaluate visceral involvement.

Treatment. Unlike Hodgkin lymphoma and most non-Hodgkin lymphoma for which standard immuno-chemotherapeutic regimens are available, there is no standard of care for MF, and its treatment depends on local expertise in the management of CTCL and drug availability, clinical staging, i.e., limited vs generalised cutaneous diseases or the absence or presence of nodal or visceral involvement, the presence of Sézary syndrome and the patient's age and fitness. In principle, **local disease** can be treated with radiotherapy or topical steroids, and **cutaneous disease without nodal or visceral diseases** can be treated with skin-directed therapy including PUVA or total skin electron beam therapy. Patients **failing skin-directed therapy or those who have nodal or visceral disease** should be treated with systemic therapy. Options for first-line systemic therapy include retinoid analogue bexarotene; single agent chemotherapy including methotrexate; interferons; or monoclonal antibody, particularly anti-CD30. Patients with Sézary syndrome should be treated with extracorporeal photopheresis (ECP). Options for second-line systemic therapy include single agent chemotherapy pralatrexate; histone deacetylase inhibitor vorinostat or romidepsin; anti-CCR4 monoclonal antibody mogamulizumab; and anti-CD52 monoclonal antibody alemtuzumab. The role of immune checkpoint inhibitor anti-PD-1 is being evaluated in clinical trial.

23.6 KEY POINTS

1. MF is the most common cutaneous T-cell lymphoma arising from CD4+ T-cells.
2. In the presence of extensive skin involvement and circulating Sézary cells, the condition is known as Sézary syndrome.
3. Local disease should be treated with radiotherapy or topical steroids. Relapsed/refractory or disseminated disease should be treated with systemic therapy.

ADDITIONAL READINGS

1. Sethi TK, Montanari F, Foss F, Reddy N. How we treat advanced stage cutaneous T-cell lymphoma—mycosis fungoides and Sézary syndrome. Br J Haematol 2021 Nov; 195(3): 352–364.
2. Whittaker S, Hoppe R, Prince HM. How I treat mycosis fungoides and Sézary syndrome. Blood 2016 Jun 23; 127(25): 3142–3153.

24 T-cell Prolymphocytic Leukaemia

24.1 CLINICAL SCENARIO

A 38-year-old man with a history of hepatitis during adolescence presented with upper right quadrant pain and dark coloured urine for 3 days. He also noticed drooling of saliva on the right side of the mouth. Physical examination showed enlarged liver and spleen at 11 and 5 cm below the costal margin, respectively. There was a lower motor neuron lesion affecting the right facial nerve.

24.2 LABORATORY REPORTS

	Results	Reference	Units
White cell count	35.6	3.9–9.9	10^9/L
Haemoglobin	14.5	13–17	g/dL
Platelet count	55	167–396	10^9/L
Alanine transaminase	424	8–58	IU/L
Alkaline phosphatase	287	42–100	IU/L
Total bilirubin	43	4–23	μmol/L
Lactate dehydrogenase	1010	118–221	IU/L
Human T-lymphotropic virus type 1	Negative	Negative	
Human immunodeficiency virus type 1 and 2	Negative	Negative	

Blood smear showed the presence of abnormal lymphoid cells, which were small with irregular nuclei, a condensed chromatin pattern and a single prominent nucleolus. Cytoplasmic blebs were evident in some cells (Figure 24.1). Flow cytometry showed that the abnormal lymphoid cells were CD3+, CD8+ and T-cell receptor (TCR) α/β+, while CD4 was negative. They also showed CD7+ and CD52+, and 30% of these were cytoplasmic TCL1 positive. Bone marrow (BM) showed extensive marrow involvement by T-cell lymphoproliferative disorder (T-LPD). The fluorescence in-situ hybridisation (FISH) for TCL1 rearrangement was positive, and *STAT5B* mutation was detected. Lumbar puncture showed a total cell count of 12×10^6/L, of which 68% were abnormal lymphoid cells.

Positron emission tomography/Computed tomography (PET/CT) showed multiple hypermetabolic lymph nodes and hepatosplenomegaly.

24.3 QUESTIONS

1. What is the likely diagnosis?
2. What is the treatment approach?
3. What is the prognosis?

24.4 CLINICAL PROGRESS

The patient was treated with anti-CD52 monoclonal antibody alemtuzumab and intrathecal methotrexate. His white cell count became normalised, and both the hepatosplenomegaly and right facial nerve palsy resolved. However, despite anti-fungal and anti-viral prophylaxis, he developed

DOI: 10.1201/9781003325413-27

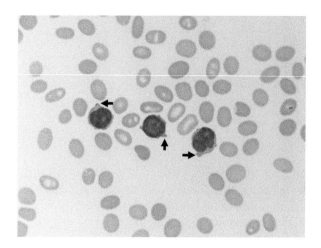

FIGURE 24.1 T-PLL cells in the peripheral blood showing the characteristic cytoplasmic blebs (Wright-Giemsa × 1000).

pneumonia by atypical *Mycobacterial haemophilum* and disseminated methicillin-sensitive *Staphylococcus aureus* (MSSA) bacteraemia, affecting the BM, skin and joints. Alemtuzumab was stopped. Four months later, his disease relapsed with abnormal circulating lymphoid cells and left facial nerve palsy. Alemtuzumab and intrathecal methotrexate were resumed. His white cells and central nervous system responded again, and he received allogeneic haematopoietic stem cell transplantation (HSCT) from his HLA-identical brother in February 2022. BM before HSCT showed residual lymphoma cells.

24.5 T-PLL

T-PLL is a rare but aggressive mature T-cell leukaemia. Most patients present with hepatosplenomegaly, generalised lymphadenopathy or skin infiltration. Anaemia and thrombocytopenia are common, and lymphocytosis > 100×10^9/L can occur rapidly. Diagnosis is based on the characteristic morphological features of abnormal circulating lymphoid cells, which are small to medium-sized, with irregular nuclei and visible nucleoli. A characteristic feature is the presence of cytoplasmic blebs. They are positive for T-cell markers including CD2, CD3, CD5, CD7 and CD52. A majority of patients are CD4+, although some patients show CD8+ or CD4 and CD8 co-expression. The most frequent chromosomal abnormality involves the inversion or translocation of chromosome 14 in which TCL1A and TCL1B (T-cell leukaemia/lymphoma) are brought into juxtaposition to the T-cell receptor (TCR) locus, leading to **TCL1A/B oncoprotein over-expression**. Mutation of genes involved in JAK/STAT signaling is commonly seen. **Loss-of-function mutations** of the tumour suppressor ataxia telangiectasia mutated (**ATM**) are also commonly encountered in T-PLL. Both aberrations cooperate to induce aberrant DNA damage response. More recently, next generation sequencing has shown recurrent **mutations of the JAK/STAT signaling** pathway, and epigenetic modifier **EZH2 and BCOR** have also been described.

24.6 MANAGEMENT

T-PLL is an aggressive T-cell leukaemia, and prompt treatment is needed. However, conventional chemotherapeutic regimens that are commonly used for lymphoma are ineffective for T-PLL. At present, anti-CD52 monoclonal antibody alemtuzumab is considered the single most active agent for this disease. Nevertheless, response is typically transient, and complications are very common, limiting its application. Allogeneic HSCT is the only curative treatment but is only suitable for young and fit patients with a suitable donor. Novel strategies based on the reactivation of p53, BCL2 and CDK targeting and inhibitors of JAK/STAT signaling are currently being tested in clinical trials.

24.7 KEY POINTS

1. T-PLL is an aggressive, mature T-cell leukaemia with characteristic morphological features and genetic aberrations.
2. Effective medical treatment for T-PLL is not available. Alemtuzumab induces transient response but is associated with significant infective complications. Allogeneic HSCT has curative potential.

ADDITIONAL READING

1. Matutes E, Catovsky D, Müller-Hermelink HK. T-cell prolymphocytic leukaemia. In: Swerdlow SH et al., eds. *WHO Classification of Tumours of Haematopoietic and Lymphoid Tissues.* International Agency for Research on Cancer 2017, pp. 346–347.

25 Hodgkin Lymphoma

25.1 CLINICAL SCENARIO

A 20-year-old woman with a history of eczema and allergic rhinitis since childhood presented with an enlarged lymph node about 2 cm in size on the left side of her neck in March 2019. Fine needle aspiration (FNA) showed suppurative inflammation, and core biopsy showed necrotising lymphadenitis. The lymph node reduced in size initially but enlarged again in May 2020 and became multiple in number. At the same time, the patient complained of generalised pruritus, night sweats and weight loss of 5 kg (usual body weight 50 kg). Excisional lymph node biopsy showed a loss of nodal architecture with **interspersed hyaline fibrotic** and lymphoid areas and several foci of necrosis. The lymphoid areas comprised a **background of inflammatory infiltrates** containing lymphocytes, plasma cells, neutrophils, eosinophils and **scattered large bi-lobed or multi-nucleated lymphoid cells** with prominent nucleoli. These abnormal lymphoid cells were positive for CD15, CD30 and Pax5 and negative for CD3 and CD20 (Figure 25.1A). Positron emission tomography/Computed tomography (PET/CT) showed multiple hypermetabolic lymph nodes in the neck, mediastinum, spleen, abdomen and pelvis (Figure 25.1B). Bone marrow examination showed no lymphoma involvement.

25.2 QUESTIONS

1. What is the diagnosis?
2. What is the treatment approach?
3. What is the prognosis?

25.3 CLINICAL PROGRESS

The patient was diagnosed classical Hodgkin lymphoma, nodular sclerosing type (cHL-NS) at Stage IIIB and received an A-AVD regimen (Adcetris [Brentuximab vedotin]- Adriamycin, Vinblastine, Dacarbazine). Her lymph nodes and pruritus resolved after 2 courses, and interim PET/CT showed a complete metabolic response. She received 4 more courses of A-AVD, and end-of-treatment PET/CT scan showed continual complete metabolic remission.

Classical Hodgkin lymphoma. Classical Hodgkin lymphoma (cHL) represents > 90% of Hodgkin lymphoma and comprises four histological subtypes, including nodular sclerosing (NS), lymphocyte-rich, mixed cellularity and lymphocyte-depleted cHL. The nodular sclerosing type accounts for > 70% cHL with peak incidence at 15–34 years. It typically affects the mediastinum and cervical lymph nodes, although abdominal and pelvic lymph nodes and the liver, spleen and bone marrow may also be involved. Histologically, the lymph nodes show a nodular pattern, with nodules surrounded by collagen bands. Necrosis may be present. Two histological features are essential in the diagnosis: **scattered large mononuclear Hodgkin cells and bi-nucleated Reed Sternberg cells** with prominent nucleoli (collectively known as HRS cells). Some HRS cells show characteristic cytoplasmic retraction, creating a "lake" around the nuclei, and are known as lacunar cells. Another diagnostic feature is the **background of non-neoplastic inflammatory cells** including small lymphocytes, eosinophils, neutrophils, histiocytes and plasma cells and fibrosis. Immunohistochemically, HRS cells are CD30+CD15+ and PAX5+, which underscores their B-cell origin. Mature B-cell surface antigen CD20 and CD79a are negative in most cases. Pan-leukocyte antigen CD45 is characteristically negative. Other cHL subtypes are uncommon and are largely defined by the cellular constituents of the inflammatory background. They are more frequently encountered in elderly populations, giving rise to the overall bimodal age distribution of cHL. Less

DOI: 10.1201/9781003325413-28

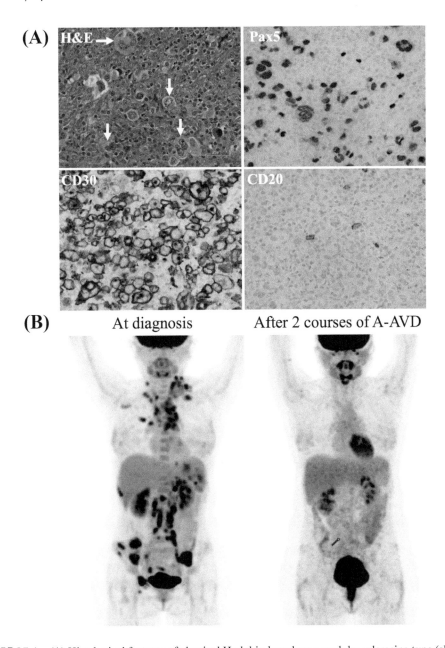

FIGURE 25.1 (A) Histological features of classical Hodgkin lymphoma, nodular sclerosing type (cHL-NS). Arrows show the pathognomonic uni-nuclear, bi-nuclear and multi-nuclear Hodgkin and Reed Sternberg (HRS) cells amidst a non-neoplastic inflammatory background comprising lymphocytes, plasma cells, neutrophils, eosinophils and hyaline fibrotic strands. (B) Treatment responses after two cycles of A-AVD (Adcetris [Brentuximab vedotin]- Adriamycin, Vinblastine, Dacarbazine), as evaluated by Positron emission tomography/Computed tomography (PET/CT) scan. (*Figure 25.1A, courtesy of Dr. Rex Au Yeung.*)

than 10% of Hodgkin lymphoma is known as nodular lymphocyte predominant Hodgkin lymphoma (NLPHL). It is distinct from cHL by the morphology and immunophenotypes of the scattered large neoplastic cells, known as lymphocyte predominant (LP) or popcorn cells, and the characteristic cellular background comprising small lymphocytes and histiocytes in a nodular meshwork of follicular dendritic cell processes.

25.4   DIFFERENTIAL DIAGNOSES

One important differential diagnosis of cHL-NS is **primary mediastinal B-cell lymphoma (PMBCL)**, a subtype of non-Hodgkin Lymphoma (NHL). Like cHL-NS, PMBCL occurs predominantly in young patients who present with mediastinal mass and cervical lymphadenopathy. Interestingly, the gene expression profile and oncogenic signals of PMBCL overlap with those of cHL-NS. The distinction between cHL-NS and PMBCL is largely histological. Specifically, PMBCL shows an abundant and diffuse rather than scattered infiltration of large atypical lymphoid cells that are mostly negative for CD15 and variable expression of CD30, and it is almost uniformly positive for surface B-cell antigen CD20 and CD79a and pan-leukocyte antigen CD45. The cellular inflammatory background is lacking in PMBCL although sclerosis is usually present. Occasionally, mediastinal lymphoma may show histological and immunophenotypic features intermediate between cHL-NS and PMBCL, which is known as "**gray zone lymphoma**". Exact diagnosis of these entities is of therapeutic and prognostic significance. Other differential diagnoses of mediastinal mass include T-lymphoblastic leukaemia/lymphoma, bronchogenic carcinoma, thymoma and mediastinal germ cell tumours.

Staging. Staging of cHL is based on the Ann Arbor Staging System and is predicated on the premise that the neoplastic cells begin in lymph nodes of one lymphatic region (Stage I), then spread along the lymphatic system to adjacent regions (Stage II) and thereafter, distribute across the diaphragm (Stage III) before they disseminate to non-lymphoid tissues (Stage IV). Patients who present with constitutional symptoms, defined by the presence of night sweats, $\geq 10\%$ body weight loss in 6 months and unexplained fever are accorded Stage B for each anatomical stage. Staging serves to guide the duration of chemotherapy and inform the prognosis of treatment.

25.5   TREATMENT AND PROGNOSIS

In general, Hodgkin lymphoma is considered a chemo-sensitive disease. Combination chemotherapy is the mainstay of treatment, with adriamycin, bleomycin, vinblastine and darcarbazine (ABVD) being the most commonly used. **Early stage disease (Stage I-IIA)** is treated by 3–4 courses of ABVD followed by involved node radiotherapy (INRT), with a view to reduce chemotherapy-related toxicity. **Advanced stage disease (Stage IIB-IV)** and patients for whom INRT is unsuitable are treated by 6 courses of ABVD. Overall, the 5-year survival of patients is above 85%.

The single most important prognostic factor is the achievement of complete metabolic response (CRm) after 2 courses of ABVD, as evaluated by PET/CT. Patients who achieve CRm would have to receive the rest of the regimen, with overall survival above 90%. Long-term toxicity of chemotherapy and radiotherapy is the main reason for treatment failure, particularly related to cardiotoxicity and secondary malignancy. Patients who fail to achieve CRm after 2 courses of ABVD would have to receive a more intensive chemotherapeutic regimen at the expense of increased myelotoxicity, secondary myelodysplastic syndrome, leukaemia and infertility. Patients who relapse after initial remission should be salvaged by alternative chemotherapeutic regimens to avoid cross-resistance. Chemo-sensitive lymphoma should be treated by myeloablative chemotherapy followed by autologous haematopoietic stem cell transplantation (HSCT).

Immunotherapy is now available for the treatment of cHL. In patients with advanced stage cHL, a combination of anti-CD30 antibody drug conjugate Brentuximab vedotin and ABVD has been shown to improve progression-free but not overall survival. Bleomycin is removed from the combination regimen as it may induce excessive pulmonary toxicity in the presence of Brentuximab. Immune checkpoint inhibitors have also been approved for the treatment of cHL that are refractory to chemotherapy or relapse after autologous HSCT. Importantly, some patients with a hitherto dismal outcome can now be salvaged by immune checkpoint inhibitors and achieve long-term remission.

Compared with other lymphoma types, Immune checkpoint inhibitors are particularly effective in cHL. RS cells show genomic amplification at 9p, resulting in over-expression of PD-L1/2 and, therefore, dependence on the immune checkpoint for tumour survival.

25.6   KEY POINTS

1. cHL-NS typically presents with cervical and mediastinal lymphadenopathy in young patients. Diagnosis depends on the presence of pathognomonic HRS cells and a non-neoplastic inflammatory background.
2. cHL-NS is generally chemo-sensitive and is highly curable. Long-term treatment toxicity, especially secondary haematological malignancy and cardiotoxicity among survivors, is a major concern.
3. Immunotherapy including immune checkpoint inhibitors and anti-CD30 antibody drug conjugate shows promising results in the treatment of newly diagnosed and relapsed and refractory cHL-NS.

ADDITIONAL READING

1. Brice P, de Kerviler E, Friedberg JW. Classical Hodgkin lymphoma. Lancet 2021; 398(10310): 1518–1527.

Plasma Cell Neoplasms

26 Amyloidosis

26.1 CLINICAL SCENARIO

A 68-year-old woman with a history of hypertension and hyperlipidaemia presented with bilateral leg swelling, facial puffiness and shortness of breath on exertion for 1 week. Physical examination confirmed ankle oedema up to the knees, and there was mild bilateral basal crepitation.

26.2 LABORATORY REPORTS

	Results	References	Units
Creatinine	54	49–82	μmol/L
Serum albumin	25	39–50	g/L
Urine Pr/Cr	1890	< 10	mg/mmol Cr
24-hr urine Pr	5.87	< 0.15	g/D
Cholesterol	9.4	< 5.2	mmol/L
Triglycerides	2.3	< 1.7	mmol/L
LDL	6.1	< 2.6	mmol/L
IgG/A/M	300/55/66	819/70/55 (LLN)	mg/dL
SPEP/Serum IFX	Negative	Negative	
Urine IFX	Negative	Negative	
Serum free κ/λ/ratio	35.8/12/2.98	19.4/26.3/1.65 (ULN)	mg/L

Pr: Protein; Cr: Creatinine; LDL: Low-density lipoprotein; SPEP: Serum protein electrophoresis; IFX: Immuonfixation; LLN: Lower limit of normal; ULN: Upper limit of normal.

Bone marrow showed no overall increase in plasma cells but the presence of CD138+ plasma cells interstitially with kappa (κ) light chain restriction. Renal biopsy was performed. The glomeruli exhibited eosinophilic, weakly PAS+ deposits in the mesangium and periphery. Periodic Schiff-Methenamine Silver (PASM) staining showed delicate spikes projecting from the outer surface of the glomerular basement membrane (GBM). Congo red staining showed salmon pink deposits in the capillary wall of the background kidney tissue (Figure 26.1A). No eosinophilic deposition was noted in the arterioles. Immunofluorescence studies showed κ light chain restriction in the mesangium. Electron microscopy (EM) showed aggregates of linear, non-branching fibrils, with each 8–10 nm in diameter (Figure 26.1B). Positron emission tomography/Computed tomography (PET/CT) scan showed no osseous lesion or lymphadenopathy.

26.3 QUESTIONS

1. What is the diagnosis?
2. What further investigations are of prognostic value?
3. What is the management?

26.4 DIAGNOSIS

The patient presented with nephrotic syndrome with serum albumin < 25 g/L and 24-hour urine protein > 3.5 g/D. The initial diagnostic clue to underlying plasma cell dyscrasia was immunoparesis,

DOI: 10.1201/9781003325413-30

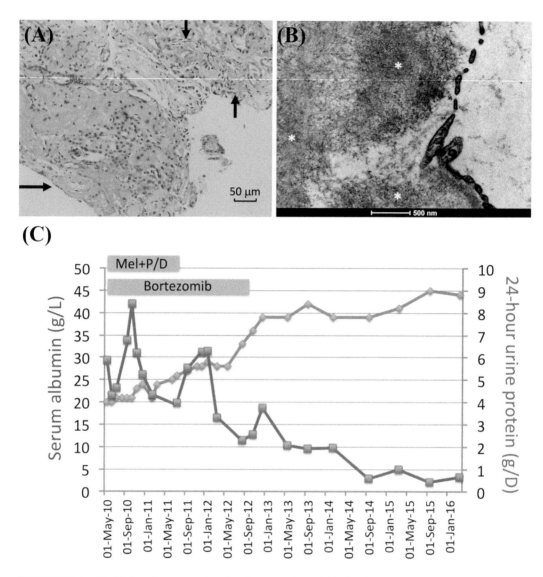

FIGURE 26.1 (A) Light microscopy showing features of amyloidosis. Congo red staining showed salmon pink (arrows) deposits in the capillary wall of the glomerulus. (B) Electron microscopic feature of renal biopsy showing the characteristic non-branching fibrils (asterisks). (C) Patient response to treatment with melphalan (mel), corticosteroid and bortezomib. P: Prednisolone; D: Dexamethasone. (*Figures 26.1A and 26.1B, courtesy of Dr. Rex Au Yeung.*)

and despite the absence of serum and urine paraproteins, there was skewing of the serum free light chain to the κ isotype. This is confirmed by bone marrow examination showing the presence of κ light chain restricted CD138+ plasma cells. Renal biopsy showed the characteristic salmon pink colour with Congo red staining, and immunostaining showed κ light chain restriction of the mesangium, and EM confirmed the presence of linear and non-branching fibrils with size characteristics of amyloid deposits. It was not multiple myeloma as there was no overall increase in plasma cells, which requires bone marrow plasma cells > 10%. The primary diagnosis was amyloid light chain amyloidosis.

26.5   AMYLOIDOSIS

Amyloidosis is a group of diseases that share in common extracellular deposition of amyloid fibril in body tissues. Fibrils were once thought to be starch-like in nature, hence the misnomer amyloid. The subtypes are distinct in aetiologies, the biochemical nature of fibrils and clinical presentations. **Amyloid light chain (AL) amyloidosis** is the most common of these diseases and is an acquired plasma cell disorder. It can occur on its own or as a complication of multiple myeloma or Waldenström macroglobulinaemia. The amyloid fibrils are made of clonal immunoglobulin light chains. It is a systemic disease primarily affecting the kidneys, but multiple organs are often involved, particularly the heart, nerves and gastrointestinal tract due to fibril deposition in different organs. **Amyloid A (AA) amyloidosis** is caused by chronic infection or inflammation, which are conditions associated with an increase in acute phase protein serum amyloid A (SAA) that deposits in tissues as amyloid fibrils. The kidneys are usually involved early in the disease course, but other organs can also be involved. **Beta-2 microglobulin amyloidosis** is seen in patients with chronic renal failure and long-term dialysis. Amyloid deposits are made of β-2 microglobulin that accumulates in tissues, particularly around joints. **Amyloid transthyretin (ATTR) amyloidosis** is caused by > 100 inherited *TTR* mutations that cause abnormal TTR protein, which deposits as amyloid fibrils. It presents after middle age, primarily with neuropathy and cardiomyopathy. Other hereditary amyloidoses are very rare. ATTR amyloidosis can also occur with wild type TTR protein, primarily in older men who present with cardiomyopathy. **Localised amyloidosis** is caused by local production of immunoglobulin light chains or other extracellular proteins. It may occur in the airway, eye or urinary bladder and usually remains as a localised disease.

26.6   CLINICAL PRESENTATION

Patients with AL amyloidosis present with a wide range of symptoms involving multiple organ systems. Kidneys are the most commonly affected, resulting in proteinuria often in the nephrotic range with ensuing hyperlipidaemia, hypogammaglobulinaemia and thrombophilic tendency. Severe cases may present with renal failure. Cardiac involvement is associated with high morbidity and mortality due to heart failure and often fatal ventricular arrhythmia. Patients with amyloid involvement of the nervous system may present with peripheral and autonomic neuropathy, and those with diffuse gastrointestinal tract involvement are at risk of diarrhoea and bleeding, which can be life-threatening. Hepatosplenomegaly and lymphadenopathy may be present. Patients may show bleeding tendency due to acquired Factor X deficiency due to its absorption by amyloid protein as well as vasculopathy due to amyloid infiltration.

26.7   INVESTIGATIONS

In patients with proteinuria, definitive diagnosis depends on renal biopsy with evidence of amyloid deposits characterised by the presence of salmon pink amorphous materials upon Congo red staining and apple green birefringence upon examination in polarised light. In the absence of these features, the typical EM feature of linear non-branching fibrils of an 8–10 nm diameter also confirms the diagnosis. Serum and urine paraproteins and/or skewing of the serum free κ/λ light chain ratio provide evidence of underlying plasma cell dyscrasia. Bone marrow examination may show amyloid involvement and the presence of clonal plasma cells. Furthermore, where the clonal plasma cells are greater than 10% or there is evidence of lymphoplasmacytic lymphoma, the diagnosis becomes AL amyloidosis complicating multiple myeloma or Waldenström macroglobulinaemia. PET/CT scan is indicated to look for evidence of skeletal lesions in myeloma, lymphadenopathy and plasmacytoma. To examine for cardiac involvement, echocardiogram and Magnetic resonance imaging (MRI) of the heart should be performed, and raised troponin and brain natriuretic peptide (BNP) are associated with inferior prognosis and severe cardiac complications. Blood pressure measurement at erect and supine positions may reveal postural hypotension due to autonomic neuropathy, and sural nerve biopsy may confirm amyloid involvement. The extent to which amyloid involvement has to be documented depends on the clinical context. Buccal mucosa, subcutaneous fat and rectal mucosa are common sites of biopsy for histological confirmation. In tertiary institutes where facilities are available, liquid chromatography/mass spectrometry (LC/MS) can be used to characterise the identity of amyloid protein for definitive diagnosis.

26.8   MANAGEMENT

Treatment should target specific organs affected by amyloidosis and the underlying plasma cell dyscrasia. For example, patients with nephrotic syndrome, angiotensin converting enzyme inhibitor (ACEI) or angiotensin renin blocker (ARB) may alleviate proteinuria, and judicious use of diuretics helps control the oedematous state. Lipid lowering agent is often needed to control hyperlipidaemia. Patients with cardiac involvement need thorough cardiology assessment, and prophylactic implantation of implantable cardioverter defibrillator (ICD) may be indicated in patients with imminent risk of fatal arrhythmia. Patients with postural hypotension due to autonomic neuropathy may improve with mineralocorticoid supplements. Treatment of underlying plasma cell dyscrasia depends on patient age and fitness. In general, the treatment approach is similar to that of multiple myeloma, with a combination of proteasome inhibitor, alkylating agent and corticosteroid being the most popular regimen that is highly effective in disease control (Figure 26.1C). More recently, anti-CD38 monoclonal antibody daratumumab has been shown to significantly enhance the efficacy of the triple therapy. In contrast, immunomodulatory agents, which are core to the treatment of multiple myeloma, are less frequently used due to a toxicity profile that is most vulnerable in the setting of AL amyloidosis, including neuropathy and renal failure. In young and otherwise fit patients, autologous haematopoietic stem cell transplantation (HSCT) may further enhance disease control. Newer agents are being evaluated for primary AL amyloidosis including anti-B-cell maturation antigen (BCMA) agent, which is used in myeloma treatment, and amyloid fibril-directed therapies, which are currently under clinical trial.

26.9   KEY POINTS

1. AL amyloidosis can affect multiple organs, but the kidneys are most frequently affected. Patients may present with severe proteinuria that causes nephrotic syndrome.
2. Tissue biopsy is essential for the diagnosis of AL amyloidosis, which shows characteristic histological features. EM may be needed in some cases.
3. Treatment of AL amyloidosis should target specific organs affected by amyloidosis and the underlying plasma cell dyscrasia.

ADDITIONAL READING

1. Bal S, Landau H. AL amyloidosis: untangling new therapies. Hematology Am Soc Hematol Educ Program 2021; 2021(1): 682–688.

27 Multiple Myeloma

27.1 CLINICAL SCENARIO

A 58-year-old woman with good past health presented after an episode of slip and fall in June 2021, resulting in back pain. Chest X-ray showed fractures of the 5th and 9th ribs and a collapsed T7 vertebra. She was otherwise well.

27.2 LABORATORY REPORTS

	Results	Reference	Units
Haemoglobin	10.1	11.7–14.9	g/dL
White cell count	6.0	3.7–9.2	10^9/L
Platelet count	265	145–370	10^9/L
Creatinine	70	49–82	μmol/L
Serum albumin	27	39–50	g/L
Serum globulin	73	24–37	g/L
Serum calcium	2.3	2.11–2.55	mmol/L
Lactate dehydrogenase	450	143–280	U/L

Blood film showed rouleaux formation and normal white cell differentials.

27.3 QUESTIONS

1. What is the next blood investigation?
2. What is the likely diagnosis?
3. What are the confirmatory investigations?
4. What is the treatment approach?

27.4 PROGRESS

The results of other investigations are as follows.

	Results	Reference	Units
IgG	510	819–1725	mg/dL
IgA	5139	70–386	mg/dL
IgM	< 20	55–307	mg/dL
β-2 microglobulin	4.99	< 1.42	μg/mL
Serum protein electrophoresis	38	Negative	g/L
Immunofixation	IgA/κ	Negative	
Serum free light chain κ/λ	195/9.5 = 20.64	κ/λ = 0.26–1.65	

The presence of skeletal abnormalities, hypergammaglobulinaemia, paraproteinaemia and immunoparesis led to the suspicion of plasma cell dyscrasia. Bone marrow (BM) examination showed an increase in plasma cells (56%) (Figure 27.1A). Flow cytometry showed that the plasma cells were

DOI: 10.1201/9781003325413-31

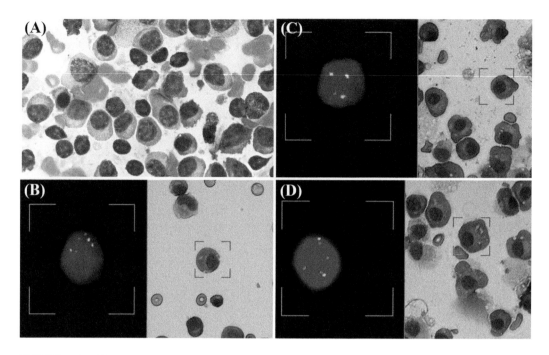

FIGURE 27.1   (A) Bone marrow smear of the patient showing an increased number of abnormal plasma cells. (Wright-Giemsa × 1000). (B–D): Interphase fluorescence in-situ hybridisation. (B) The left panel showed trisomy 5 of the index plasma cell (right panel) with three orange signals (representing 5q31) and three green signals (representing 5p15.2). (C) The left panel showed t(4;14) by locus-specific IGH/FGFR3 Dual Colour Dual Fusion probe. Key: Orange (O) signal: FGFR3 (4p16); green (G) signal: IGH (14q32); yellow (F) signal: IGH-FGFR3 fusion. The presence of the typical 1G1O2F pattern confirmed t(4;14) translocation of the index plasma cells in the right panel. (D) Detection of 1q21 gain by CKS1B/CDKN2C (P18) Amplification/Deletion probe. Key: Red signal: CKS1B (1q21); Green signal: CDKN2C (1p32.3). The left panel showed 1q21 gain (4 instead of 2 copies) of the index plasma cell in the right panel.

positive for CD138 and CD38 with cytoplasmic κ light chain restriction. Cytogenetics were normal 46, XX. Fluorescence in-situ hybridisation (FISH) of plasma cells that were selected based on CD138 expression showed the presence of t(4;14) translocation that involved IgH/FGFR3, a gain of 1q21 and trisomy 5 (Figure 27.1B–27.1D, left panels). Skeletal survey showed a collapsed L1, multiple lytic lesions in both upper femurs, proximal humeri, skull vault, ischium and pubic bone. Positron emission tomography/Computed tomography (PET/CT) scan confirmed diffuse lytic lesions in the axial skeleton with pathological fractures and vertebral collapses (Figure 27.2A).

27.5   TREATMENT PROGRESS

The patient received a combination of daratumumab, bortezomib (Velcade), lenalidomide (Revlimid) and dexamethasone (Dara-VRd) for 4 courses and bisphosphonate every 4 weeks. She had to wear a corset and took an opioid painkiller for pain control. In January 2022, she received high-dose melphalan treatment followed by autologous haematopoietic stem cell transplantation (HSCT), which has been uneventful. She has received further treatment with Dara-VRd as post-HSCT consolidation, followed by lenalidomide maintenance. At the time of writing, she remained in complete remission and was asymptomatic (Figure 27.2B).

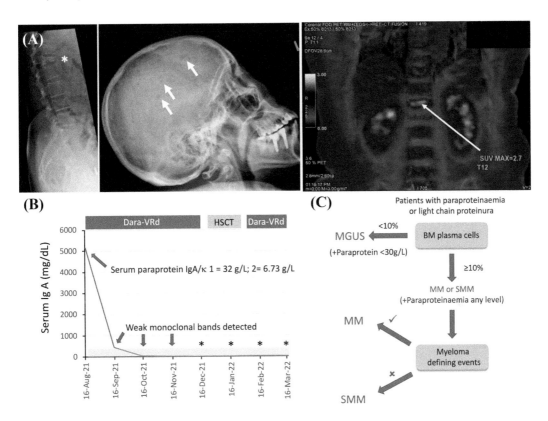

FIGURE 27.2 (A) X-ray showed L1 collapse (left) and lytic lesions in the skull vault (left right), and Positron emission tomography/Computed tomography (PET/CT) scan showed metabolic uptake in the vertebrae, particularly at the T12 level (right). (B) Serum IgA and paraprotein responses to myeloma treatment. The asterisks denote no monoclonal protein detectable. The grey area at the bottom shows the normal reference range for serum IgA (70–386 mg/dL). Dara-VRd: Daratumumab, bortezomib (Velcade), lenalidomide (Revlimid) and dexamethasone; HSCT: Haematopoietic stem cell transplantation. (C) Diagnostic algorithm of multiple myeloma (MM), smoldering MM (SMM) and monoclonal gammopathy of unknown significance (MGUS). BM: Bone marrow. SMM also includes cases with BM plasma cells < 10% but serum paraprotein ≥ 30 g/L.

27.6   MULTIPLE MYELOMA

Multiple myeloma (MM) is a multifocal neoplastic disease of plasma cells characterised by an increased number of morphologically **abnormal plasma cells** (> 10% of BM cells), the presence of **paraproteins** in serum and/or urine and evidence of **organ damage**. It is a disease of the elderly with a median age of onset of 70 years, and > 90% of patients are older than 50 years. Subtypes of MM are defined by the isotype of the paraproteins as follows (Table 27.1).

TABLE 27.1
Prevalence of myeloma subtypes

Isotype	Percentage
IgG	50%
IgA	20%
Light chain	20%
IgD or non-secretary	< 10%

27.7   PATHOGENESIS

MM is an indolent disease, and most patients would have antecedent monoclonal gammopathy of unknown significance (MGUS) and a stage of smoldering MM before progression to overt and symptomatic MM. The pathogenesis involves intrinsic cell changes and induction of microenvironmental changes conducive to oncogenesis. The initial oncogenic transformation entails chromosomal gains or translocation involving IgH (see the following) and occurs in a post-germinal centre B-cell or plasma cell, giving rise to MGUS. Subsequent genetic and epigenetic changes confer survival advantage to the expanding neoplastic clones. Furthermore, they induce structural changes in the extracellular matrix, functional changes of BM stromal cells, activation of angiogenesis and remodeling of the bone structure. Collectively, they create a pro-oncogenic microenvironment that is conducive to the survival and expansion of neoplastic plasma cells.

27.8   CLINICAL FEATURES

Clinical features are manifestations of end organ damage as a result of the neoplastic plasma cells in the acronym "**CRAB**" that entails hyper**c**alcaemia due to bone resorption, **r**enal insufficiency due to tubular damage by excess light chain, hypercalcaemia or direct plasma cell infiltration, **a**naemia due to marrow failure or chronic renal insufficiency and **b**one involvement due to plasma cell deposition. In addition, patients may also present with **extramedullary deposition** of plasma cells known as plasmacytoma, neuropathy and spinal cord compression because of encroaching plasmacytoma or vertebral fracture, **amyloid light chain (AL) amyloidosis**, opportunistic infection due to **immunoparesis** that usually occurs in advanced diseases or **bleeding** as a result of thrombocytopenia or Factor Xa depletion due to its absorption by amyloid. Occasionally, hitherto asymptomatic patients may present with abnormal serum globulin (either an increase or decrease) or rouleaux formation in blood smear.

27.9   INVESTIGATIONS

To confirm the diagnosis, initial investigations should include serum protein electrophoresis and immunofixation, serum free light chain and urine protein electrophoresis. If positive for monoclonal proteins, then BM aspiration and biopsy should be performed. Neoplastic plasma cells are characterised by the presence of multi-nucleated and immature nuclei with dispersed chromatin and prominent nucleoli and expression of CD138 and CD38 using flow cytometry and immunohistochemistry. Demonstration of clonality based on monotypic light chain expression, i.e., predominant expression of one light chain type over the other, is essential. More than 90% of patients show karyotypic abnormalities, mostly detectable by FISH. Conventional karyotyping is less sensitive. Patients presenting with significant proteinuria should have renal biopsy to confirm the presence of amyloid. Conventional skeletal survey based on X-ray of the axial skeleton and appendages is now superseded by computed tomography (CT) that shows much higher sensitivity for bone lesions. Both PET/CT or low-dose whole body CT scan are widely used for the evaluation of bone lesions and detection of lymphoproliferative disease in patients presenting with paraproteinaemia.

27.10   PROGNOSTICATION

In the past, MM prognoses were defined not only by the Durie-Salmon system based on the severity of CRAB and disease load but also by the International Staging System (ISS) based on serum β-2 microglobulin and albumin levels. These systems are now superseded by the **Revised ISS** that takes into consideration β-2 microglobulin and albumin as in the ISS, plus additional factors including serum lactate dehydrogenase (LDH) and the presence of high-risk chromosomal abnormalities detectable by FISH, i.e., del(17p), t(4;14) and t(14;16). The Mayo Stratification of Myeloma and Risk-Adapted Therapy (mSMART) uses more risk-defining cytogenetic abnormalities and a gene expression profile and proliferative index of plasma cells, which are not available in most laboratories, to identify the subgroup of patients with inferior prognosis.

27.11   MANAGEMENT APPROACH

At present, MM is considered an incurable disease. However, new therapies have emerged that have substantially improved patient outcomes. Patients with MGUS may progress to overt MM at 1% per year and therefore need close monitoring but not active treatment (Figure 27.2C). It is important to clinically distinguish overt MM that requires treatment from smoldering myeloma that does not based on the presence of "myeloma defining events" including the aforementioned CRAB, clonal plasma cells ≥ 60% in BM, skewing of the serum κ/λ ratio ≥ 100 folds and ≥ 1 BM lesions of 5 mm or more in MRI. The management of MM entails the following aspects.

Emergency management. MM patients presenting with cord compression due to plasmacytoma or vertebral fracture need urgent surgical decompression to prevent permanent neurological debility. Those with hypercalcaemia should be treated with hydration, bisphosphonate and steroids. Renal failure patients may benefit from temporary dialysis before the effects of myeloma-specific therapy set in.

Myeloma therapy. The major classes of drugs that are now available for myeloma treatments are shown in Table 27.2.

Myeloma treatment has undergone rapid changes in recent decades that generally have resulted in improved outcomes. Patients with newly diagnosed MM are treated with **combination regimens** comprising 3–4 drugs of different mechanistic classes. After 4 courses, transplant eligible patients may receive **autologous HSCT**, followed by maintenance therapy. Selected patients with features associated with high relapse risk may benefit from post-HSCT consolidation before maintenance therapy. Autologous HSCT is not curative but has been shown to improve progression-free survival of these patients. In transplant ineligible patients, combination regimens used for initial treatment should continue until disease progression. More recently, **chimeric antigen receptor T-cell** therapy targeting B-cell maturation antigen (BCMA) on the myeloma cell surface has been shown to be highly effective for refractory cases.

Myeloma bone diseases. Patients with extensive skeletal involvement by myeloma should receive regular bisphosphonate therapy for bone protection, at least for the first 12 months of MM diagnosis. Bisphosphonates attach to hydroxyapatite binding sites on the bone surface and can enter osteoclasts and disrupt their functions during bone resorption. Denosumab, a monoclonal antibody

---

TABLE 27.2

Classes of Drugs Used for the Treatment of Multiple Myeloma

Mechanisms	Examples
Proteasome inhibitor	Bortezomib, Carfilzomib, Ixazomib
Immunomodulatory agents	Lenalidomide, thalidomide, Pomalidomide
Alkylating agents	Cyclophosphamide, melphalan, bendamustine
Corticosteroids	Dexamethasone, prednisolone
Monoclonal antibody	
Naked antibody	Daratumumab (CD38), Isatuximab (CD38), Elotuzumab (SLAMF7)
Bi-specific T-cell engager	Teclistamab-cqyv (BCMA x CD3)
Antibody drug conjugate	Belantamab mefodotin (BCMA) (withdrawn)
Nuclear export inhibitor	Selinexor
Histone deacetylase inhibitor	Panobinostat

against receptor activator of NFκB ligand (RANKL) that blocks osteoclast function and reduces bone resorption, can also be considered for MM bone disease, especially for patients with renal impairment in whom bisphosphonate usage is more limited. Patients with imminent fracture of long bones or vertebral instability may receive prophylactic surgery. Adequate analgesics should be ensured at all times.

27.12   KEY POINTS

1. Symptomatic MM is characterised by the presence of neoplastic plasma cells in BM (> 10% of BM cells), paraproteins in serum and/or urine and evidence of organ damage.
2. Symptomatic MM is thought to evolve from antecedent MGUS and smoldering MM. Patients with symptomatic MM need treatment. MGUS and smoldering MM should be monitored.
3. There has been substantial improvement in treatment options and patient outcomes in MM in recent decades. A comprehensive approach should be adopted. However, MM is still considered an incurable disease.

ADDITIONAL READINGS

1. van Nieuwenhuijzen N, Spaan I, Raymakers R, Peperzak V. From MGUS to multiple myeloma, a paradigm for clonal evolution of premalignant cells. Cancer Res 2018; 78(10): 2449–2456.
2. Bal S, Giri S, Godby KN, Costa LJ. New regimens and directions in the management of newly diagnosed multiple myeloma. Am J Hematol 2021; 96(3): 367–378.
3. McKenna RW, Kyle RA, Kuehl WM et al. Plasma cell neoplasms. In: Swerdlow SH et al., eds. *WHO Classification of Tumours of Haematopoietic and Lymphoid Tissues.* International Agency for Research on Cancer 2017, pp. 243–248.

28 POEMS Syndrome

28.1 CLINICAL SCENARIO

A 49-year-old woman with hyperlipidaemia presented with a 1-year history of numbness of both lower limbs from the feet to mid-shin. Nerve conduction velocity (NCV) showed generalised axonal polyneuropathy with demyelination. Blood tests for autoimmunity, tumour markers, paraneoplastic markers and heavy metal levels were unremarkable. Cerebrospinal fluid (CSF) was acellular, and protein was 0.96 g/L (normal range: 0.15–0.6), suggesting cytoalbumin dissociation. The patient was followed up in the clinic for symptom monitoring.

Two years later, she complained of progressive and distal weakness of her lower limbs, resulting in bilateral footdrop, and she had to walk with a frame. She also complained of dusky colour changes of her lower limbs. She was given prednisolone, azathioprine and 2 courses of intravenous immunoglobulin to no avail. Physical examination showed plethora and hepatomegaly 2 cm below the costal margin. Fundoscopy showed bilateral optic disc swelling.

28.2 LABORATORY REPORTS

	Results	Reference Range	Units
Haemoglobin	16.5	11.5–14.8	g/dL
White cell count	7.69	3.89–9.93	10^9/L
Platelet count	460	167–396	10^9/L

Liver and renal function tests: Unremarkable.
Blood film: Normal. Mild thrombocytosis.

28.3 QUESTIONS

1. What are the abnormalities?
2. What is the likely diagnosis?
3. What are the next investigations?
4. What is the treatment approach?

28.4 POEMS SYNDROME

In this patient, unexplained polyneuropathy, polycythaemia, thrombocytosis, hepatomegaly, papilloedema and skin changes suggested a diagnosis of POEMS syndrome, *viz.*, **p**olyneuropathy, **o**rganomegaly, **e**ndocrinology, **m**onoclonal protein and **s**kin changes. Serum protein electrophoresis (SPEP) was negative for monoclonal protein. However, urine protein electrophoresis showed a free monoclonal lambda light chain. Serum free lambda light chain was modestly elevated at 33.2 (5.71–26.30 mg/L), with a normal free lambda to kappa light chain ratio. The plasma level of vascular endothelial growth factor (VEGF) was 2615 pg/mL (Cut-off: 200 pg/mL). Positron emission tomography/Computed tomography scan showed several tiny osteosclerotic foci at the L2, L4, left sacrum, pelvis, right proximal humerus and left femoral head with no discernible fluorodeoxyglucose (FDG) hypermetabolic activity (Figures 28.1A and 28.1B). There was no evidence of lymphadenopathy. Bone marrow aspirate showed a marked increase in megakaryocytes, and some were

DOI: 10.1201/9781003325413-32

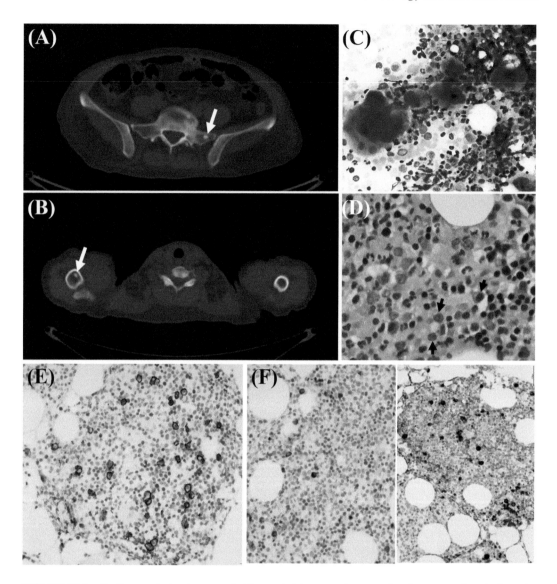

FIGURE 28.1 Positron emission tomography/Computed tomography scan showing osteosclerotic focus in the left sacrum (A) and right humerus (B) (arrows). (C) Marked megakaryocytic hyperplasia and large hyperlobulated megakaryocytes (Wright-Giemsa × 1000). (D) Trephine biopsy showing a patchy increase in plasma cells (H&E × 400). (E) Immunohistochemistry study by CD138 highlights the plasma cells (× 200). (F) The plasma cells showing lambda light chain restriction (× 200). Left panel: Lack of kappa light chain expression; Right panel: presence of lambda light chain expression. (*Figures 28.1C–28.1F, courtesy of Dr. Albert Sin.*)

large and hyperlobulated (Figures 28.1C and 28.1D). Trephine showed patchy infiltrate of abnormal plasma cells, which were CD138+ and lambda light chain restricted (Figures 28.1E and 28.1F).

POEMS syndrome is a rare paraneoplastic syndrome arising from underlying plasma cell dyscrasia. The pathogenesis of POEMS syndrome is currently unclear but is thought to be related to recurrent mutations in the neoplastic plasma cells and increased proinflammatory and angiogenic factors in the tumour microenvironment. POEMS syndrome comprises a constellation of signs and symptoms, with peripheral neuropathy and the presence of plasma cell dyscrasia being mandatory for diagnosis (Table 28.1).[1] Peripheral neuropathy, presented with numbness of the limbs, is the

---

TABLE 28.1

POEMS Syndrome Diagnostic Criteria

Mandatory

Demyelinating polyneuropathy

Monoclonal plasma cell disorder

Major

Sclerotic bone lesions

Elevated vascular endothelial growth factor (VEGF)

Castleman disease

Minor

Extravascular volume overload

Organomegaly

Endocrinopathy

Skin changes

Papilloedema

Polycythaemia and thrombocytosis

---

predominant symptom that may evolve over time to produce motor deficits. Cranial nerve involvement and dysautonomia are exceedingly rare. Given the similarity to chronic inflammatory demyelinating polyradiculoneuropathy (CIDP), all patients suspected of CIDP should be assessed for POEMS before treatment or when conventional treatment is ineffective. Unlike myeloma, plasma cell dyscrasia in POEMS is of a low tumour load, requiring a high index of suspicion. SPEP may be normal, and urine protein electrophoresis and serum free light chain are more sensitive. An increase in bone marrow plasma cells may be subtle, and immunohistochemistry for CD138, which denotes plasma cells and the demonstration of light chain restriction, is needed. Lambda light chain restriction is demonstrable in over 95% of POEMS cases. Sclerotic bone lesions, in contrast to osteolytic lesions in multiple myeloma, are present in 95% of patients.

Other features of POEMS are diverse. Endocrinopathies have occurred in a large majority of patients with POEMS, with hypogonadism being the most common. Diabetes mellitus and hypothyroidism are also commonly seen. Skin manifestations are variable, including hyperpigmentation, haemangiomata, hypertrichosis, vascular skin changes (acrocyanosis and Raynaud's phenomenon) and fingernail changes (white nails and clubbing). Extravascular volume overload may occur, presenting with peripheral oedema, ascites or pleural effusion. Papilloedema, which is often asymptomatic, is a common occurrence. An elevated plasma VEGF level is of diagnostic value and can be used to monitor disease progress. POEMS syndrome is also associated with arterial and venous thromboses due to an increase in multiple procoagulants.

28.5 PATIENT PROGRESS

The patient was treated with a combination of bortezomib (Velcade), lenalidomide (Revlimid) and dexamethasone (VRd). Autologous haematopoietic stem cell transplantation (HSCT) was offered to the patient but was declined. Two years later, she developed carcinoma of the left breast, which was treated by mastectomy. There was no evidence of metastasis. Since then, she has been treated with bortezomib monotherapy as maintenance for nearly 4 years. Her lower limb numbness and weakness have both improved, and she can walk unaided. Serum free light chain level was normalised, and urine protein electrophoresis has become negative.

28.6 TREATMENT

As most patients present with progressive neuropathy, early diagnosis of POEMS syndrome is critical to mitigate the hitherto relentless clinical debility. The treatment goal is eradication of the neoplastic plasma cell clone, thereby halting the progression of clinical diseases, particularly the debilitating motor deficits. Given the thrombophilic state, prophylactic anti-coagulation should be considered in patients with active POEMS syndrome. **In patients with localised disease**, i.e., < 3 bone lesions and no demonstrable clonal plasma cells in bone marrow, localised radiotherapy should be given. Relief of symptoms may take months to years, with neuropathy being the slowest to respond. **Patients with systemic disease**, i.e., ≥ 3 bone lesions or the presence of clonal plasma cells in marrow, should receive systemic therapy. Upfront high-dose melphalan followed by autologous HSCT have been the mainstays of treatment and result in a clinical response in most patients, but most patients eventually relapse. Patients ineligible for autologous HSCT should receive a multi-agent regimen akin to multiple myeloma. This entails various combinations of an immunomodulatory agent, proteasome inhibitor, corticosteroid, alkylating agent and more recently, anti-CD38 monoclonal antibody in settings of newly diagnosed and relapsed or refractory POEMS syndrome. In most cases, triple or quadruple therapies have been shown to induce effective clinical responses, and with continuous treatment, the responses are durable. Whether autologous HSCT could be replaced by a non-transplantation approach would have to be formally addressed.

28.7 KEY POINTS

1. Patients with unexplained polyneuropathy should be investigated for underlying plasma cell neoplasm for the diagnosis of POEMS syndrome.
2. Early diagnosis and treatment may mitigate the hitherto relentless clinical debility.
3. The treatment goal is the eradication of the neoplastic plasma cell clone.

ADDITIONAL READING

1. Khouri J, Nakashima M, Wong S. Update on the diagnosis and treatment of POEMS (polyneuropathy, organomegaly, endocrinopathy, monoclonal gammopathy, and skin changes) syndrome: a review. JAMA Oncol 2021; 7(9): 1383–1391.

Thalassaemia and Haemoglobin Disorders

29 Beta Thalassaemia Major

29.1 CLINICAL SCENARIO

A 49-year-old woman with transfusion-dependent thalassaemia came for medical follow up. She was married with no children. She has been regularly transfused since childhood, requiring 2 units of packed cells every 4 weeks. Splenectomy was performed at age 20 years. She has also been regularly receiving subcutaneous deferoxamine and oral deferiprone with additional deferasirox since 2014. Her elder sister and parents were known to have the thalassaemia trait. She has a short stature and prominent cheek (Figure 29.1A).

29.2 LABORATORY REPORTS

	Results	References	Units
Haemoglobin	8.4	11.7–14.8	g/dL
Mean corpuscular volume	77.9	82–96	fL
Mean corpuscular haemoglobin	25.5	27.5–33.2	pg
White cell count	10.44	4.4–10.1	10^9/L
Platelet count	607	17–380	10^9/L
Alkaline phosphatase	76	32–93	U/L
Alanine aminotransferase	103	7–37	U/L
Aspartate aminotransferase	56	14–30	U/L

Blood film showed hypochromic microcytic red cells, marked anisopoikilocytosis and post-splenectomy changes and was characterised by the presence of target cells, Howell Jolly bodies and circulating nucleated red cells (Figure 29.1B).

29.3 QUESTIONS

1. What is the clinical condition?
2. What are the complications?
3. What is the management plan and prognosis?

29.4 CLINICAL PROGRESS

The patient was diagnosed beta thalassaemia major, also known as Cooley's anaemia. She developed hepatitis C virus (HCV) infection during childhood with elevated alanine aminotransferase (ALT) (Genotype Ib) and was on regular monitoring until 2017 when she received a 24-week treatment with direct anti-viral agents daclatasvir and asunaprevir with a clearance of serum HCV-RNA. In addition, she had primary amenorrhoea, requiring hormonal replacement therapy, and developed osteoporosis and primary hypothyroidism at age 30 years on bisphosphonate and thyroxine replacement. She was diabetic and required oral hypoglycaemic agents. Furthermore, her compliance with iron chelation was unsatisfactory, and her serum ferritin level was persistently raised, ranging from 10,000 to 30,000 pmol/L. Magnetic resonance imaging (MRI) T2* in 2020 showed a T2* relaxation time of myocardium of 13.1 milliseconds, and that of the liver was 1.14 milliseconds, which suggests severe iron overloading of the heart and liver.

DOI: 10.1201/9781003325413-34

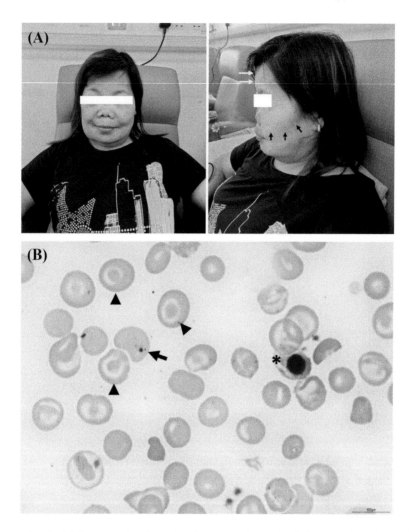

FIGURE 29.1 (A) Facial features of patient, showing a prominent cheek (arrows). (B) Blood film (Wright-Giemsa × 1000) showing the presence of nucleated red cells (asterisk), target cells (arrowheads) and Howell Jolly body (arrow). (*Figure 1A, courtesy of Dr. Gloria Hwang.*)

29.5 BETA THALASSAEMIA

Genetics. Beta thalassaemia is an autosomal recessive disorder characterised by defective production of β globin chains. More than 350 mutations in the β globin gene have been identified, which are mostly single nucleotide substitution or small indels (insertions or deletions) within the β globin gene or its immediate flanking sequence. Unlike alpha thalassaemia, gross deletion of the β globin gene is rare. Mutations leading to a complete absence of β globin production are denoted as β^0, whereas mutations leading to reduced production are denoted as β^+. Beta thalassaemia is most prevalent in the Mediterranean, South East Asian and Middle East regions, where malaria is endemic. The prevalence in Europe and North America is increasing due to immigration.

Genetic modifiers. Clinical severity of beta thalassaemia is modified genetically. For instance, co-existing alpha thalassaemia reduces chain synthesis and ameliorates the imbalance between globin chains and, therefore, the clinical severity. Persistent expression of fetal haemoglobin (HbF) ($\alpha_2\gamma_2$) due to an increase in BCL11A expression is associated with the milder phenotype. Co-existing haemoglobinopathy, notably HbE, which has a high prevalence in South East Asia, may also modify the phenotype (see the following).

Clinical features. Traditionally, beta thalassaemia is classified by genotype and clinical severity. Homozygous β^0 (beta thalassaemia major, also known as Cooley's anaemia) shows the most severe phenotype, as it is transfusion-dependent from early on in life. Compound heterozygous β^0/β^+ may develop beta thalassaemia major or intermedia. Beta thalassaemia intermedia tends to present later in life with mild to moderate anaemia. However, exacerbation of anaemia may occur during pregnancy, intercurrent viral infection or surgery. Heterozygous β/β^0 or β/β^+ shows the beta thalassaemia trait, with very mild and asymptomatic anaemia. More recently, patients are classified based on their transfusion requirement. In transfusion-dependent thalassaemia (TDT), patients require life-long and regular transfusion for survival. These cases are mainly beta thalassaemia major or severe HbE–beta thalassaemia. In non-transfusion-dependent thalassaemia (NTDT), patients require no or only occasional transfusion. These cases include thalassaemia intermedia or mild or moderate HbE–beta thalassaemia.

Diagnosis. The initial suspicion of beta thalassaemia arises from hypochromic microcytic anaemia and the personal and family history of anaemia and cholelithiasis. Intercurrent iron deficiency, which is also associated with hypochromic microcytic anaemia, has to be ruled out. Diagnosis of beta thalassaemia is confirmed by the increase in haemoglobin A_2 (HbA$_2$) and HbF by using electrophoresis or high-performance liquid chromatography (HPLC). These features were masked in our patient due to regular blood transfusion. In cases with normal HbA$_2$ and HbF, alpha thalassaemia should be ruled out by the detection of haemoglobin H (HbH) inclusion bodies and immunochromatography.

29.6 COMPLICATIONS

Complications arise from the key **clinicopathologic changes** of beta thalassaemia, namely, ineffective erythropoiesis, including chronic anaemia and haemolysis and the **side-effects of chronic red cell transfusion**. Important examples are listed as follows.

Chronic anaemia. Chronic anaemia in paediatric patients may lead to a delay in development and growth retardation. The associated marrow expansion and extramedullary haematopoiesis may lead to skeletal deformity including protruding maxilla and frontal bossing, giving rise to the characteristic morphologic appearance in these patients. Other features of extramedullary haematopoiesis include hepatosplenomegaly and paravertebral pseudotumour.

Iron overload. Iron overload is a major complication arising from life-long transfusion and increased iron absorption secondary to ineffective erythropoiesis and the suppression of hepcidin synthesis in the liver. Excessive iron load leads to the saturation of transferrin binding capacity and non-transferrin-bound iron deposition in major organs including the heart, liver and endocrine organs, which causes cardiotoxicity, liver cirrhosis, hypogonadism, hypothyroidism and diabetes mellitus. Before the era of effective iron chelation, cardiac arrythmia due to iron deposition was a major cause of mortality in patients with thalassaemia major.

Infection. Chronic iron overload in thalassaemia may induce infection by siderophilic bacteria including the Yersinia and Klebsiella species. Iron chelator deferoxamine may aggravate this infection by making circulating iron more accessible to these bacteria. Splenectomised patients are at risk of infection by encapsulated bacteria including *Streptococcus pneumoniae*, *Haemophilus influenzae* and *Neisseria meningitidis*. Before nucleic acid testing (NAT) was widely available in transfusion medicine, viral infections including human immunodeficiency virus (HIV), HCV and hepatitis B virus (HBV) and their sequelae were the major causes of morbidity and mortality in chronically transfused patients.

Hyperbilirubinaemia and cholelithiasis. Chronic haemolysis and the ensuing unconjugated hyperbilirubinaemia enhance the formation of pigmented gallstones. Symptomatic patients require cholecystectomy.

Thrombosis. Chronic haemolysis is associated with increased risks of venous and occasionally, arterial thrombosis due to alteration of the red cell membrane and platelet activation.

Recurrent thromboembolism in the pulmonary circulation can lead to pulmonary hypertension. Cerebrovascular events may also occur.

Osteopenia and osteoporosis. Loss of bone mineral density can result from compensatory marrow expansion, hypogonadism due to iron overload and toxicity of iron chelators.

29.7   MANAGEMENT

Prenatal counselling of prospective mothers who are carriers of the beta thalassaemia trait is essential, and screening of partners for the trait is needed to inform patients of the risk of developing homozygous beta thalassaemia, particularly TDT. In patients with TDT, regular transfusion is the mainstay of treatment with a target Hb of 9–10 g/dL. Iron chelation should begin when serum ferritin reaches 1000 ng/mL or when 10 units of red cells have been transfused. Deferoxamine, given subcutaneously or intravenously, has been the standard treatment but is inconvenient for patients, which limits compliance. Two oral iron chelators, deferiprone and deferasirox, have been licensed. They can be used as monotherapy or deferiprone can be used in combination with deferoxamine to reduce iron load. More recently, luspatercept, an activin receptor ligand trap that blocks SMAD2/3 signaling and enhances erythroid maturation, has been approved to reduce the transfusion requirement in TDT. In selected TDT patients, allogeneic haematopoietic stem cell transplantation (HSCT) is considered a curative therapeutic option. Clinical trials of gene therapy are currently underway that entail the collection of haematopoietic stem cells from patients with TDT and viral transduction *ex vivo* to introduce exogenous beta-like globin or disruption of BCL11A to induce increase in HbF that can ameliorate anaemia. In NTDT, the Hb level and iron load status should be monitored. Iron chelation may be needed in patients with excessive iron overload.

29.8   KEY POINTS

1. Beta thalassaemia results from defective production of the β globin chain. In beta thalassaemia major, patients require life-long transfusion from childhood.
2. Complications of beta thalassaemia major arise from chronic anaemia and haemolysis, thrombophilia and iron overloading due to chronic blood transfusion. Effective iron chelation is important to avoid cardiac, liver and endocrine complications.
3. Blood transfusion and allogeneic HSCT are the mainstays of treatment. Recently, luspatercept has also been approved. Gene therapy is under clinical trial and may improve the outcome of these patients.

ADDITIONAL READINGS

1. Taher AT, Musallam KM, Capellini MD. Beta thalassaemias. New Engl J Med 2021; 384: 727–743.
2. So JCC, Ma ESK. Hemoglobin and hemoglobinopathies. In: Rifai N, Chiu RWK, Young I et al., eds. *Tietz Textbook of Laboratory Medicine*. 7th Edition. Elsevier 2022, Ch. 77.

30 Haemoglobin H Disease

30.1 CLINICAL SCENARIO

A 30-year-old woman presented with malaise for two months, following an episode of upper respiratory tract infection. She was married but had no children. She had cholecystectomy at the age of 20 years. Her mother and elder sister have always been pale-looking and had gallstones. Both underwent cholecystectomy at about 30 years old. The patient was also pale, and there was splenomegaly about 2 fingerbreadths below the costal margin. She never had blood transfusion before.

30.2 LABORATORY REPORTS AT PRESENTATION

	Results	References	Units
Haemoglobin	5.9	11.7–14.8	g/dL
Mean corpuscular volume	74	82–96	fL
Mean corpuscular haemoglobin	20.9	27.5–33.2	pg
White cell count	3.24	4.4–10.1	10^9/L
Platelet count	136	17–380	10^9/L
Lactate dehydrogenase	340	100–250	IU/L
Total bilirubin	60	7–19	mmol/L

Blood film showed microcytosis, hypochromia, anisocytosis and the presence of target cells (Figure 30.1).

30.3 QUESTIONS

1. Suggest one initial biochemical and one haematological investigation.
2. What is the likely diagnosis?
3. What is the management plan?

30.4 CLINICAL PROGRESS

Further laboratory investigations are as follows.

	Results	References	Units
Ferritin	1400	34–337	pmol/L
Haemoglobin A_2	0.9	2.3–3.0	%
Fetal haemoglobin	< 0.30	< 0.90	%
Haemoglobin H inclusion	98		%
Genotype	Southeast Asian (SEA) deletion/haemoglobin Quong Sze (Hb QS) double heterozygous		

The patient has become transfusion-dependent since the first presentation, requiring 2–3 units of packed cells every 2 months. Splenectomy was performed in December 2014, and her haemoglobin (Hb) has become stable at 8–9 g/dL without transfusion. She developed pulmonary embolism in July 2015 and has been receiving rivaroxaban since then.

DOI: 10.1201/9781003325413-35

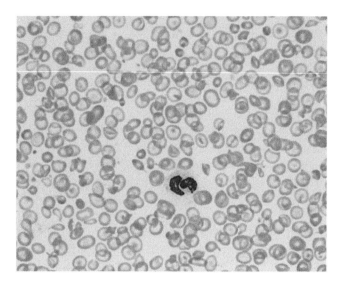

FIGURE 30.1   Peripheral blood smear of deletional haemoglobin H (HbH) disease (Wright-Giemsa × 1000) showing microcytosis, hypochromia, anisocytosis and the presence of target cells.

30.5   THALASSAEMIA SYNDROMES

Haemoglobin disorders are a group of diseases characterised by pathological defects in globin chain synthesis. They comprise diseases with a quantitative globin chain defect including α and β thalassaemia, those with qualitative defect, i.e., haemoglobinopathy (or structural Hb variants) and those with hereditary persistence of fetal Hb (HbF). Their co-occurrence gives rise to a wide spectrum of thalassaemia syndromes and related diseases. Currently, thalassaemia is categorised by the need for life-long transfusion. Patients with **non-transfusion-dependent thalassaemia** are not dependent on transfusion for survival, but anaemia can be exacerbated during physical stress and illness or can become progressive. This includes most cases of HbH disease, β thalassaemia intermedia and HbE/β thalassaemia. Patients with **transfusion-dependent thalassaemia** require life-long transfusion since early in life. This includes β thalassaemia major, severe cases of HbE/β thalassaemia and severe and very often non-deletional forms of HbH disease. The presence of thalassaemia is thought to protect patients from severe malaria and is prevalent in areas where malaria is endemic, including Southeast Asia, the Mediterranean, the Indian subcontinent, the Middle East, and Africa.

30.6   PATHOGENESIS OF HAEMOGLOBIN H DISEASE

Haemoglobin is a tetramer comprising 2 alpha or alpha-like (zeta) globin chains and two beta or beta-like (delta, gamma and epsilon) globin chains. Genes encoding for α and γ chains are duplicated (αα/αα, γγ/γγ), and there are two copies of each gene in each allele. Gene encoding for β chain is single in each allele (β/β). In fetus, Hb is made up of two α and two γ chains (α2γ2) termed HbF or fetal Hb. After birth and in infancy, γ chain is switched to β chain, and Hb consists of two α and β chains (α2β2) termed HbA or adult Hb. In α thalassaemia, defective α chain production results in formation of γ4 tetramers, also known as Hb Barts in the fetal stage and β4 tetramers, called HbH, in adults. Both γ4 and β4 tetramers show very high oxygen affinity, and their failure to offload oxygen results in tissue hypoxia. β4 tetramer is unstable, causing haemolytic anaemia.

HbH disease belongs to the family of α thalassaemia and is predominantly characterised by deletion or less commonly, non-deletional mutations of 3 out of 4 copies of α globin genes. The various forms of mutations give rise to variable disease severities. In Southeast Asia, a DNA deletion of chromosome 16 that **removes both α globin genes** occurs (--^{SEA}) in 5% of the population, resulting in α^0 thalassaemia carrier (deletion of 2 α globin genes *in cis*). In contrast, smaller deletions result in the **removal of a single α globin gene** (α$^+$ thalassaemia carrier), with -α$^{3.7}$ (removal of 3.7 kb) being the most common, which occurs in up to 70–90% of the populations in Melanesia and Nepal. Apart from gene deletions, non-deletional α globin gene mutations also occur and may result in HbH disease when co-inherited with the Southeast Asian (SEA) deletion. In fact, the non-deletion form of HbH disease often gives rise to clinically more profound anaemia and iron overload, splenomegaly, haemolysis and thrombosis. The common non-deletion mutation in Southeast Asia is known as Hb Constant Spring, in which mutation of the stop codon results in extension of α globin by 31 amino acids, which is produced in a very low amount due to mRNA instability. Another non-deletion mutation Hb Quong Sze results in mutated α globin that is unable to assemble in stable tetramers and is rapidly degraded. Disruption of 4 copies of α globin genes gives rise to hydrops fetalis, and 1 or 2 copies can have normal Hb or mild hypochromic microcytic anaemia.

30.7 CLINICAL PRESENTATIONS

Depending on the underlying genetic aberration, HbH disease shows variable severity and presentations, ranging from being asymptomatic to symptomatic anaemia during intercurrent infection or progressive transfusion dependence. Some patients may present with complications including gallstones, chronic leg ulcers and splenomegaly. A chronic haemolytic state also confers thrombophilic tendency. A family history of anaemia and chronic haemolysis, manifesting as biliary stones and cholecystitis, supports the diagnosis.

30.8 LABORATORY FINDINGS

Typical blood smear of HbH disease shows microcytosis, hypochromia, anisopoikilocytosis (variation in cell size and shape) and the presence of target cells and nucleated red blood cells. Iron deficiency anaemia should be ruled out. The Hb pattern shows a low HbA2 (α2δ2) level and the presence of HbH (β4). Incubation of red cells with mild oxidants such as brilliant cresyl blue results in formation of HbH precipitates known as HbH inclusion bodies. The ferritin level is often raised, even in patients who have not begun transfusion, resulting from increased iron absorption, a condition known as non-transfusion-dependent iron overload.

30.9 DIFFERENTIAL DIAGNOSIS

With family history, characteristic laboratory findings and clinical features, HbH disease should be readily diagnosed. A peculiar differential diagnosis is acquired HbH disease, which is mostly associated with myelodysplastic syndrome (MDS) and myeloproliferative neoplasm (MPN). The causative mechanism is unclear, but there is significant down-regulation of α globin gene expression possibly due to somatic mutations of the *ATRX* gene or acquired deletion of chromosome 16p. Despite the presence of hypochromic microcytic red cells, anisopoikilocytosis and the presence of HbH inclusions, acquired HbH disease can be distinguished from HbH disease by the lack of family history, elderly age of onset and evidence of MDS or MPN. In addition, HbH disease can be associated with mental retardation due to ATR-16 syndrome in which extended deletions (1–2 Mb) of chromosome 16p remove both α globin genes; it can also be associated with another form with a complex phenotype including hypertelorism, a flat nasal bridge, a triangular upturned nose, a wide mouth, genital abnormalities and severe mental retardation due to mutations in the *ATRX* gene.

30.10   MANAGEMENT

Management of HbH disease depends on its clinical severity. Patients with mild HbH disease are clinically well and do not require treatment. Patients should be warned of disease exacerbation due to intercurrent infection and to avoid oxidising agents. Those with profound and symptomatic anaemia should receive blood transfusion, and their iron status should be closely monitored. Patients with splenomegaly may receive splenectomy while considering the risk of thrombosis. Premarital screening of a spouse for the thalassaemia trait is important for the prevention of stillbirth due to hydrops fetalis.

30.11   KEY POINTS

1. HbH disease belongs to the family of non-transfusion-dependent α thalassaemia with a high prevalence in Southeast Asia.
2. Haematological features entail hypochromic microcytic anaemia, reduced HbA_2, the presence of HbH (β4) and HbH inclusion in red cells upon brilliant cresyl blue staining.
3. HbH disease results from a deletion (more common, milder disease) or non-deletion mutation (less common, more severe disease) or their combination, which affects 3 out of 4 α globin genes.
4. The different combinations of deletion or non-deletion mutation in a particular patient result in variable clinical severity from being asymptomatic to the severe phenotype of anaemia, haemolysis, splenomegaly and thrombosis.

ADDITIONAL READINGS

1. Galanello R, Cao A. Alpha-thalassemia. Genet Med 2011; 13(2): 83–88.
2. Viprakasit V, Ekwattanakit S. Clinical classification, screening and diagnosis for thalassemia. Hematol Oncol Clin N Am 2018; 32: 193–211.
3. Piel FB, Weatherall DJ. The A-thalassemias. N Engl J Med 2014; 371: 1908–1916.
4. So JCC, Ma ESK. Hemoglobin and hemoglobinopathies. In: Rifai N, Chiu RWK, Young I et al., eds. *Tietz Textbook of Laboratory Medicine.* 7th Edition. Elsevier 2022, Ch. 77.

31 Sickle Cell Disease

31.1 CLINICAL SCENARIO

A 40-year-old woman from West Africa came to Hong Kong as a foreign diplomat. Her baseline haemoglobin was 5–6 g/dL, and she had repeated pain episodes in her childhood and teenage years. She started taking hydroxyurea 6 years ago and has been free of pain since then. She was admitted to hospital for bilateral lower limb swelling and pain for 1 week and had fever, vomiting and diarrhoea 5 days before the onset of this episode. She was a single child, and her patients were apparently asymptomatic.

31.2 LABORATORY REPORTS

	Results	References	Units
Haemoglobin	3.9	11.7–14.8	g/dL
Mean corpuscular volume	90.3	82–96	fL
White cell count	13.9	4.4–10.1	10^9/L
Platelet count	738	17–380	10^9/L
Lactate dehydrogenase	637	100–250	IU/L
Total bilirubin	18	7–19	mmol/L

Blood film showed red cells with sickle shape, target cells, slight polychromasia and giant platelets (Figure 31.1A).

31.3 QUESTIONS

1. What is the likely diagnosis?
2. What are the confirmatory tests?
3. What is the management plan?

31.4 CLINICAL PROGRESS

Haemoglobin (Hb) analyses were performed as follows.

	Results	References	Units
Fetal haemoglobin	10.1	< 1.0	%
Haemoglobin A2	4.1	2.5–3.4	%
Haemoglobin H bodies	Negative	Negative	
Acid electrophoresis	Abnormal	Normal	
Alkaline electrophoresis	Abnormal	Normal	

Comment: On high-performance liquid chromatography (HPLC), no HbA was detected. A variant band (85%) was eluted in the S window. The Hb variant migrated to the "S" position in acid and alkaline electrophoresis. The findings were consistent with homozygous HbS (Hb SS).

DOI: 10.1201/9781003325413-36

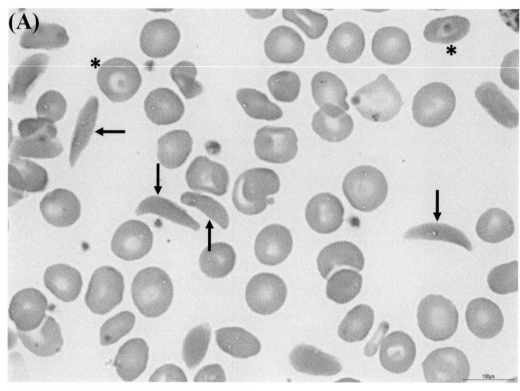

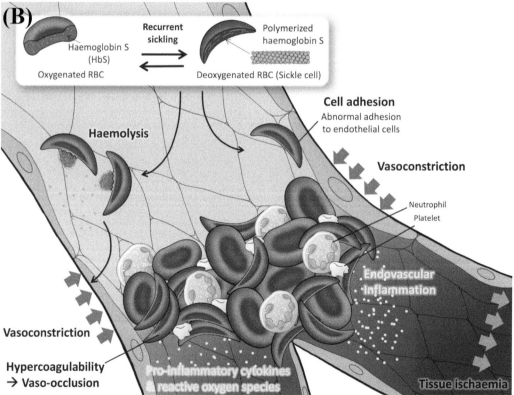

FIGURE 31.1 (A) Red cells with sickle shape (arrows), target cells (asterisks) and slight polychromasia in sickle cell anaemia (Wright-Giemsa × 1000). (B) Pathogenesis of sickle cell disease.

31.5   SICKLE CELL DISEASE

Sickle cell disease (SCD) results from the inheritance of sickle Hb (HbS) in the homozygous state (Hb SS) or double heterozygous state with other Hb variants such as Hb C (Hb SC) or β thalassaemia (HbSβ). HbS results from a single gene mutation of the β globin chain in which glutamate is substituted by valine at position 6 (HBB E6V). SCD is prevalent in sub-Saharan Africa, the Mediterranean basin, the Middle East and India, where patients with sickle cell trait (SCT) are protected from severe forms of malaria. However, due to international travel, SCD may be encountered in different geographical areas.

31.6   PATHOGENESIS

SCD results from polymerisation of the deoxygenated Hb carrying HbS, leading to distortion of red blood cells into a sickle shape, hence the name sickle cells. These sickle cells show increased expression of adhesion molecules, which causes abnormal adhesion to endothelial cells and their dysfunction. The cascade of molecular and cellular events results in a wide range of pathological consequences including haemolysis, endovascular inflammation, hypercoagulability and vaso-occlusion, causing tissue ischaemia (Figure 31.1B). SCD patients show a wide variation in clinical manifestations and severities due to the presence of co-existing genetic modifiers, e.g., the α thalassaemia trait and endogenous fetal Hb (HbF) levels, and non-genetic modifiers, e.g., climate, air quality and socioeconomic factors.

31.7   MANAGEMENT

Management of SCD entails the prevention of sickling crises, treatment of acute pain episodes and management of complications arising from recurrent sickling crises. A multi-disciplinary approach is needed.

31.8   PREVENTION OF SICKLING CRISES

Early treatment is beneficial to avoid long-term complications. For decades, **hydroxyurea** was the only therapy available for such treatment. It is a ribonucleotide reductase inhibitor that induces production of HbF. HbF inhibits HbS polymerisation, the initiating pathogenetic event in red cell sickling. More recently, L-glutamine, crizanlizumab and voxelotor have also been approved. **Oral L-glutamine** has been shown to decrease reactive oxygen species (ROS) in red blood cells to reduce their sickling and adhesion. **Crizanlizumab** is a monoclonal antibody targeting P-selectin on activated platelet and endothelial cells, reducing vaso-occlusion. **Voxelotor** promotes binding of HbS to oxygen, hence reducing HbS polymerisation. For severe cases, allogeneic haematopoietic stem cell transplantation should be considered. Gene therapy for SCD is being tested in clinical trials.

31.9   ACUTE SICKLING CRISES AND THEIR MANAGEMENT

Patients presenting with **severe pain episodes** should be managed with adequate analgesics including parenteral opioids and non-steroidal anti-inflammatory agents. In patients who present with pleuritic chest pain, fever, hypoxaemia or tachypnoea and chest X-ray infiltrates, **acute chest syndrome** should be considered and treated with packed cell transfusion or exchange transfusion. SCD patients show functional asplenia and are susceptible to **infection**; they should also be treated empirically as such until proven otherwise. Patients presenting with neurological deficits should be investigated as **ischaemic stroke** resulting from the blockade of major cerebral vessels and should receive exchange transfusion as guided by the HbS level, in addition to standard stroke therapy. **Anaemia exacerbation** may be secondary to splenic sequestration when patients present with left upper quadrant pain due to splenomegaly or aplastic crisis precipitated notably by Parvovirus B19 and other viral infections. Urgent blood transfusion is warranted. **Biliary stones** result from a chronic haemolytic state and should be managed accordingly. **Priapism**, defined by a painful erection of more than 4 hours, should be treated with supportive measures failing which surgical intervention, as exemplified by local injection of sympathomimetics or corporal aspiration, should be considered. **Venous thromboembolism (VTE)** is common in SCD and should be treated by anticoagulation.

31.10   CHRONIC SICKLE CELL DISEASES AND THEIR MANAGEMENT

Patients with **chronic pain** should be managed by adequate analgesics and when necessary, antidepressants and cognitive behavioural therapy. **Avascular necrosis** resulting from bone ischaemia should be handled in collaboration with orthopaedic surgeons, and in severe cases, arthroplasty may be needed. **Retinopathy** is common, which results from retinal ischaemia and secondary neovascularisation and haemorrhage. Regular ophthalmological assessment is essential, and photocoagulation laser therapy may be needed. **Nephropathy**, due to sickling and ischaemia in renal medulla, hence glomerular and tubular damage, may present with albuminuria and may be managed by angiotensin-converting enzyme inhibitor. **Leg ulcers** result from the vaso-occlusin of skin particularly in areas over bony prominence. In severe cases, patients should be referred to a special wound care unit. **Pulmonary hypertension** results from chronic thromboembolic events and endothelial cell damage during recurrent sickling. Effective treatment is lacking for this condition, and patients should be referred to cardiology specialist care.

31.11   KEY POINTS

1. SCD is caused by homozygous HbSS or double heterozygous HbS and other prevalent Hb variants.
2. HbS polymerisation and red cell sickling are central to the pathogenesis of SCD, leading to haemolysis, endovascular inflammation, hypercoagulability, vaso-occlusion and tissue ischaemia.
3. Management focuses on the prevention and treatment of acute and recurrent sickling crises.

ADDITIONAL READING

1. Kavanagh PL, Fasipe TA, Wun T. Sickle cell disease. JAMA 2022; 328(1): 57–68.

32 Methaemoglobinaemia

32.1 CLINICAL SCENARIO

A 30-year-old woman was admitted to an intensive care unit (ICU) for confusion. She took 15 tablets of dapsone (1500 mg), which was prescribed for her underlying dermatitis herpetiformis, 1 hour before admission after a quarrel with her husband. She was markedly cyanosed upon admission and was given a rebreathing mask. Her oxygen saturation was 90%.

32.2 LABORATORY REPORTS

	Results	Reference	Units
pH	7.49	7.35–7.45	
Partial pressure of oxygen	16.6	10.6–14.0	kPa
Partial pressure of carbon dioxide	4.1	4.7–6.0	kPa
Bicarbonate	23	22–26	mmol/L
White cell count	7.0	3.89–9.93	10^9/L
Haemoglobin	11.2	11.5–14.8	g/dL
Platelet count	241	167–396	10^9/L

Urine toxicology: Dapsone present.
Biochemistry and clotting profile were normal.

32.3 QUESTIONS

1. Why is there a discrepancy between low oxygen saturation by pulse oximetry and a normal partial pressure of oxygen in arterial blood (PaO_2) in the blood gas sample?
2. What is the reason for the patient's confusion?
3. What is the clinical problem?

32.4 CLINICAL PROGRESS

The presence of severe cyanosis, occurrence of dapsone overdose and presence of a saturation gap, i.e., discrepancy between low oxygen saturation by pulse oximetry and a normal PaO_2 in the blood gas sample, suggested a diagnosis of methaemoglobinaemia.

32.5 LABORATORY REPORTS

	Results	Reference	Units
Methaemoglobin	52.1	0–0.5	%
Carboxyhaemoglobin	1.3	0–3	%

The patient received 2 doses of intravenous methylene blue treatment in the first 24 hours with an initial response, followed by a rebound shortly thereafter. Subsequently, she received intravenous

DOI: 10.1201/9781003325413-37

infusion of methylene blue over the next 2 days, and her plasma methaemoglobin level became nearly undetectable (Figure 32.1A). Clinically, her confusion has resolved, and she became asymptomatic.

32.6   NORMAL OXYGEN TRANSFER IN HAEMOGLOBIN

Under physiological conditions, deoxyhaemoglobin (deoxyHb) contains ferrous iron in its heme moiety (Figure 32.1B). In pulmonary circulation, deoxyHb combines with oxygen to form oxyhaemoglobin (oxyHb) with iron in a ferric superoxide anion complex. In peripheral tissue, oxyHb offloads

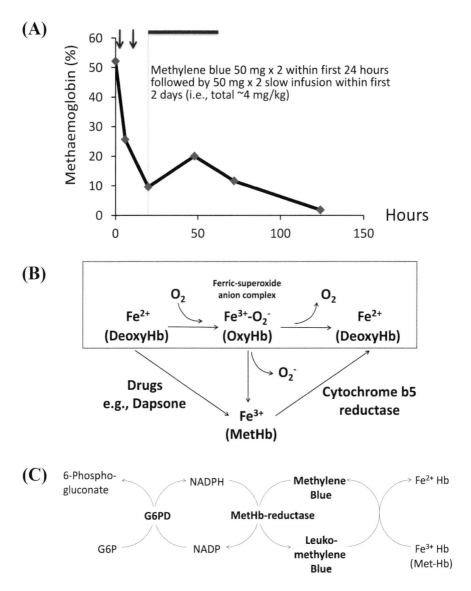

FIGURE 32.1   (A) Response of the methaemoglobin level to methylene blue. (B) Pathogenesis of methaemoglobinaemia. The red box indicates normal oxygen transfer. DeoxyHb: Deoxyhaemoglobin; OxyHb: Oxyhaemoglobin; MetHb: Methaemoglobin. (C) Biochemical pathway highlighting the therapeutic mechanism of methylene blue and the importance of glucose-6-phosphate dehydrogenase (G6PD). The G6PD level must be checked in patients before methylene blue treatment. G6P: Glucose-6-phosphate; NADP: Nicotinamide adenine dinucleotide phosphate; NADPH: Reduced form of NADP; Hb: Haemoglobin.

oxygen (O_2) and returns to the deoxyHb state. Rarely, it releases oxygen anion (O_2^-) to become methaemoglobin (MetHb) that contains ferric iron. MetHb is normally converted to deoxyHb by cytochrome b5 reductase. In its physiological state, MetHb occurs at 0–0.5% of total Hb. However, upon exposure to oxidising agents, e.g., dapsone, deoxyHb can be oxidised directly to MetHb. Alternately, defective cytochrome b5 reductase can hamper reduction of MetHb to deoxyHb. In these circumstances, the MetHb level increases. MetHb does not bind oxygen. Moreover, in its presence, oxygen affinity of deoxyHb in the tetramer is increased. As a result, MetHb shifts the oxygen dissociation curve to the left, causing tissue hypoxia.

32.7   DRAWBACK OF PULSE OXIMETRY IN METHAEMOGLOBINAEMIA

Pulse oximetry is generally used to evaluate patients with cyanosis and respiratory distress. It differentiates oxyHb from deoxyHb based on their differential absorbance at 2 wavelengths of light (660 nm and 940 nm). The ratio of light absorption at each wavelength is converted into oxygen saturation (SpO_2). MetHb generates optical interference and increases light absorption at both wavelengths. SpO_2 becomes falsely low at a low MetHb level and falsely high at a high MetHb level. In fact, at a very high MetHb level, SpO_2 becomes saturated at around 85%. As a result, SpO_2 does not reflect cyanosis and tissue hypoxia in methaemoglobinaemia.

32.8   SATURATION GAP

Saturation gap refers to a low SpO_2 measured by pulse oximetry despite a normal oxygen saturation measured by arterial blood gas (ABG). The partial pressure of oxygen (PO_2) in ABG measurement reflects plasma oxygen content but not the oxygen-carrying capacity of haemoglobin (Hb) and is normal in methaemoglobinaemia even when cyanosis and tissue hypoxia are clinically apparent. The presence of a saturation gap should raise a suspicion of methaemoglobinaemia.

32.9   CAUSES OF METHAEMOGLOBINAEMIA

Methaemoglobinaemia can be hereditary and acquired. Hereditary causes are rare and are due to cytochrome b5 reductase deficiency and a genetic variant of Hb that is predisposed to formation of MetHb (haemoglobin M disease). Acquired causes are more common and are mostly due to exogenous agents (Table 32.1).

32.10   CLINICAL PRESENTATION

The clinical presentation depends on the level of MetHb. At MetHb ≤ 20%, patients are usually asymptomatic, although some patients may show cyanosis. Above > 20%, patients become

TABLE 32.1
Examples of Drugs Causing Methaemoglobinaemia

Classes	Drugs (examples)
Nitrates	Nitroglyercin, nitroprusside
Local anaesthetics	Benzocaine, lidocaine
Antibiotics	Dapsone
Anti-Malarials	Chloroquine, primaquine
Industrial/Household agents	Aniline dyes, Naphthalene

symptomatic, reflecting tissue hypoxia. These symptoms include headache, dizziness and weakness, and electrocardiogram may show sinus tachycardia. At MetHb above 50%, patients may develop seizure, coma, lactic acidosis, myocardial ischaemia and arrhythmia. A MetHb level > 70% is incompatible with life.

32.11 TREATMENT

Treatment depends on the level of MetHb, presence of symptoms and underlying causes. Hereditary methaemoglobinaemia is rare, and when it occurs, it is usually mild; avoidance of exposure to precipitating agents may suffice. Acquired methaemoglobinaemia is mostly due to drugs and exposure to exogenous agents, which should be stopped immediately. The goal should be elimination of the incriminating agents, for instance, by gastric lavage and activated charcoal absorption. For symptomatic patients, treatment should aim at rapid reduction of the MetHb level. Intravenous methylene blue is used (Figure 32.1C). It is converted to leuko-methylene blue as NADPH is converted to NADP. Leuko-methylene blue reduces MetHb to ferrous deoxyHb. However, NADP is reduced back to NADPH as G6P is converted to 6-phospho-gluconate, a process that requires G6PD. For dapsone-induced methaemoglobinaemia, prolonged treatment may be required due to the prolonged elimination half-life of dapsone because of enterohepatic circulation. In patients with coexisting G6PD deficiency, methylene blue cannot reduce MetHb and instead induces oxidation damage to red blood cells, causing oxidative haemolysis. In these patients, ascorbic acid, exchange transfusion or hyperbaric oxygen should be considered.

32.12 KEY POINTS

1. Methaemoglobinaemia is a medical emergency.
2. Clinical suspicion arises from exposure of causative agents, dark colour of the blood sample, marked cyanosis and the saturation gap between SpO_2 and PaO_2 in the blood gas sample.
3. Methylene blue is the mainstay of treatment. Repeated dosing is often required.

ADDITIONAL READING

1. Iolascon A, Bianchi P, Andolfo I et al. SWG of red cell and iron of EHA and EuroBloodNet: recommendations for diagnosis and treatment of methemoglobinemia. Am J Hematol 2021; 96(12): 1666–1678.

Nutritional and Aplastic Anaemia

33 Aplastic Anaemia

33.1 CLINICAL SCENARIO

A 36-year-old woman with good past health presented with heavy menstruation, easy bruising and progressive shortness of breath for 2 weeks. There was no family history of blood diseases or malignancies. She was pale, and there were bruises on her upper limbs.

33.2 LABORATORY REPORTS

	Results	References	Units
Haemoglobin	4.9	11.5–14.8	g/dL
White cell count	2.56	3.89–9.93	10^9/L
Platelet count	4	167–396	10^9/L
Neutrophil count	0.3	2.01–7.74	10^9/L
Reticulocyte count	0.5	0.5–2.5	%

Liver and renal function tests were normal. Blood film showed no abnormal circulating cells.

Bone marrow (BM) was markedly hypocellular (20%) for age with a slight prominence of normal lymphocytes. Cytogenetic analysis showed normal karyotype.

33.3 QUESTIONS

1. What are the next investigations?
2. What is the diagnosis?
3. What are the potential causes?
4. What is the management approach?

33.4 INVESTIGATIONS

Examination of blood film is essential to rule out abnormal red cell morphology, dysplastic neutrophils and the presence of abnormal circulating cells. Initial investigations for hitherto unexplained pancytopenia should include a history of exposure to chemotherapeutic agents and irradiation and family history of haematological diseases and recent infections, particularly of hepatitis virus that has been associated with immune-mediated aplastic anaemia (AA). Physical examination is mostly negative in AA patients, but morphologic abnormalities should raise the suspicion of syndromal diseases causing inherited bone marrow failure (BMF). Meanwhile, lymphadenopathy or organomegaly should be further investigated for large granular lymphocyte leukaemia (LGLL) that is also associated with immune-mediated BMF. The presence of LGL should prompt further investigation for LGLL. Flow cytometry should be performed to screen for paroxysmal nocturnal haemoglobinuria (PNH) and test for defective DNA repair based on *in vitro* exposure to diepoxybutane (DEB) for Fanconi anaemia. BM examination is essential to confirm hypocellularity and rule out abnormal cellular infiltration. Karyotypic analysis is needed to identify changes typical of myelodysplastic syndrome (MDS) and to detect mutations characteristic of MDS or acquired AA, which help confirm diagnosis.

DOI: 10.1201/9781003325413-39

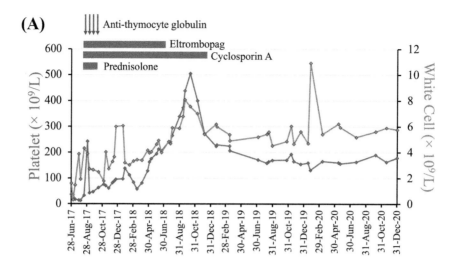

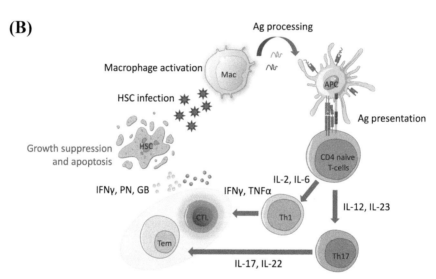

FIGURE 33.1 (A) Haematological response to immunosuppression in this severe aplastic anemia (AA) patient. (B) Proposed pathogenesis of severe AA. Mac: Macrophage; Ag: Antigen; APC: Antigen-presenting cell; CTL: Cytotoxic T-lymphocyte; Tem: Effector memory T-lymphocyte; Th: T helper cell; IFNγ: Interferon gamma; PN: Perforin; GB: Granzyme B; TNFα: Tumour necrosis factor alpha; IL: Interleukin; HSC: Haematopoietic stem cell.

33.5 CLINICAL PROGRESS

Flow cytometry of peripheral blood showed small populations of glycosylphosphatidylinositol (GPI)-deficient monocytes, neutrophils and red blood cells, consistent with a small PNH clone. Next generation sequencing (NGS) showed only *BCOR1* mutation. Serology for hepatitis B virus and hepatitis C virus was non-reactive. A diagnosis of severe AA was made. The patient was treated with anti-thymocyte globulin (ATG), cyclosporin A, corticosteroid and eltrombopag. Her haematological parameters improved after 4 months and reached normal levels after 12 months of treatment (Figure 33.1A). Cyclosporin A and eltrombopag were stopped after 18 and 12 months, respectively.

33.6   APLASTIC ANAEMIA

This patient suffered from AA, which can be categorised into very severe, severe and moderate AA based on the severity and number of blood lineages affected. Pathologically, AA is characterised by the lack of normal haematopoietic cells in blood or bone marrow rather than the presence of abnormal cells. Patients develop pancytopenia, and haematopoietic cells in the bone marrow are characteristically replaced by fat. AA belongs to the spectrum of bone marrow failure (BMF) syndromes, which based on pathophysiology, can be iatrogenic, resulting from exposure to chemo-irradiation or toxins; inherited due to germline mutations of the genes involved in DNA repair, telomere maintenance, haematopoiesis and immune checkpoints; and immune-mediated, which is initiated by immune attack against haematopoietic progenitor cells. BMF syndromes include AA, hypoplastic MDS, LGLL and PNH.

33.7   PATHOPHYSIOLOGY

AA is thought to arise from prior infection of haematopoietic stem cells (HSC), leading to macrophage activation and phagocytosis of either the pathogens or components released by infected HSC (Figure 33.1B). Macrophages migrate to the lymph nodes and present antigen to antigen-presenting cells (APC) and then to naïve CD4+ T-cells. These T-cells differentiate into T helper (Th) 1 cells that release interferon gamma (IFNγ) and Tumour necrosis factor alpha (TNFα) to activate CD8+ cytotoxic T-lymphocyte (CTL) and macrophages. The response aims to remove the infected cells, but in AA, it targets HSC and inhibits HSC growth either directly by inducing apoptosis by direct granzyme B and perforin release or indirectly by paracrine inhibitory effects of IFNγ, TNFα and Fas ligand. If the autoimmune process persists, then naïve CD4+ T-cells may differentiate into the Th17 phenotype via interleukin (IL)-23 and IL-12 stimulation. Th17 cells induce selection of oligoclonal effector memory CD8+ T-cells that sustain growth suppression and apoptosis of HSC. They also reduce the function and number of regulatory T-cells (Treg). The immunologic basis of AA is clinically evident. In 10–15% of cases, haematopoietic cells show a 6p loss of heterozygosity, representing escape clones that survive autoimmunity-targeting human leukocyte antigen alleles. Similarly, clonal expansion of PNH cells is also evident, which suggests selection for haematopoietic cells that are deficient in GPI-anchored proteins due to acquired mutation of phosphatidylinositol glycan class A (*PIGA*) in HSC.

33.8   DIFFERENTIAL DIAGNOSIS

Hypoplastic MDS (hMDS) is a major differential diagnosis of AA. Conventionally, MDS is characterised by cytopenia and BM hypercellularity, which is attributed to ineffective haematopoiesis. On the contrary, hMDS is characterised by marrow hypocellularity, a high response rate to immunosuppressive therapy and favourable prognosis. hMDS can be distinguished from AA by a number of features. For demographics, AA occurs more commonly in young patients with a female preponderance, whereas hMDS is mostly a disease of the elderly. Pathologically, hMDS is characterised by dysplastic megakaryocytic and granulocytic lineages, an increase in blasts and occasionally, marrow fibrosis, which are features hitherto absent in AA. Moreover, BM from AA patients typically shows a normal karyotype, except for the loss of sex chromosomes, which is considered benign in nature, while pathogenic cytogenetic changes are more often seen in hMDS. Genetically, somatic mutations associated with conventional MDS are more commonly seen in hMDS than AA, except for *BCOR/BCORL1* mutations, which are not infrequently seen in AA. Furthermore, the presence of PNH clones is more suggestive of AA rather than hMDS. All of these distinguishing features should be considered in the differential diagnosis of AA.

33.9   MANAGEMENT APPROACH

Management of AA depends on its severity. Patients with mild AA who do not require transfusion can be observed to evaluate the rate of progression. Patients with profound cytopenia who are transfusion-dependent should receive prompt treatment. Young patients with suitable HSC donors should receive upfront allogeneic haematopoietic stem cell transplantation (HSCT), which is associated with a high success rate. Patients without HSC donors or those who are unfit and ineligible for HSCT should receive immunosuppressive therapy that comprises anti-thymocyte globulin, cyclosporin A and corticosteroid. More recently, addition of thrombopoietin mimetics to this regimen has been shown to improve response and reduce relapse, resulting in better treatment outcomes.

33.10   KEY POINTS

1. AA is thought to arise from HSC infection and its subsequent growth suppression and apoptosis induced by immune activation.
2. AA is characterised by the absence of abnormal cells in blood and BM. hMDS is a major differential diagnosis.
3. Treatment of AA depends on its severity and entails immunosuppression and allogeneic HSCT.

ADDITIONAL READINGS

1. Durrani J, Maciejewski JP. Idiopathic aplastic anemia vs hypocellular myelodysplastic syndrome. Hematology Am Soc Hematol Educ Program 2019; 2019(1): 97–104.
2. Bono E, McLornan D, Travaglino E. Clinical, histopathological and molecular characterization of hypoplastic myelodysplastic syndrome. Leukemia 2019; 33: 2495–2505.
3. Young NS. Aplastic anemia. New Engl J Med 2018; 379: 1643–1656.
4. Giudice V, Selleri C. Aplastic anemia: pathophysiology. Semin Hematol 2022; 59: 13–20.

34 Iron Deficiency Anaemia

34.1 CLINICAL SCENARIO

A 45-year-old woman with good past health presented with shortness of breath upon exertion for the past 3 months. She used to jog for at least 5 km almost every day, and now she had to stop a few times in the middle of her jog to catch a breath. At rest, she could feel her heart bounding forcefully and frequently. She thought the symptoms were due to her imminent menopause and took some herbal supplements without avail. Her menstruation has been regular and normal in flow and her bowel opening and stool have been unremarkable. She was single and had never smoked or drunk.

34.2 LABORATORY RESULTS

	Results	Reference Range	Units
Haemoglobin	6.9	11.5–14.8	g/dL
Mean corpuscular volume	63.6	82.0–95.5	fL
Mean corpuscular haemoglobin	17.7	27.0–32.4	pg
Mean corpuscular haemoglobin concentration	27.8	32.1–34.9	g/dL
White cell count	5.07	3.89–9.93	10^9/L
Platelet count	479	167–396	10^9/L
Serum iron	1.7	6.6–26	mmol/L
Total iron binding capacity	87.4	44.8–80.6	mmol/L
Transferrin saturation	2	15–45	%

34.3 QUESTIONS

1. What are the haematologic abnormalities?
2. What are the potential causes?
3. What is the treatment approach?

34.4 IRON METABOLISM

Iron is predominantly stored as haemoglobin (Hb) in erythroid cells in both their precursor and mature forms in bone marrow (BM) and circulation, where more than two-thirds of the iron content in the body is stored. The other sites of iron store include hepatocytes, BM macrophages and to a lesser extent, skeletal muscle, where iron is stored as myoglobin. Macrophage phagocytose senescent red cells and recycle iron by releasing ferric iron for Hb synthesis. Therefore, the iron cycle for Hb synthesis is almost a closed loop, with most of the iron needed for Hb synthesis being derived from senescent red cells (about 20 mg daily), and the contribution of dietary iron absorption is minimal (about 1 mg daily). Iron absorption and utilisation are regulated by a hormone known as hepcidin. Specifically, BM erythroid precursors, known as erythroblasts, express transferrin receptors (TFR) on their surface and take up diferric iron-bound transferrin, the main iron carrier protein

DOI: 10.1201/9781003325413-40

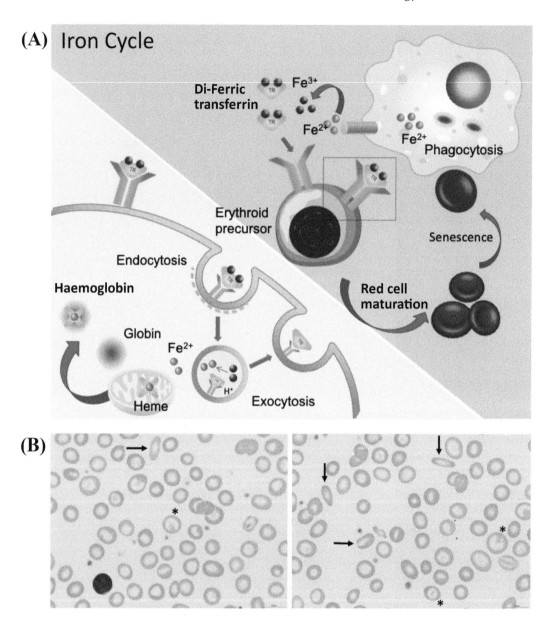

FIGURE 34.1   (A) Iron cycle forms nearly a closed loop in the generation of haemoglobin. (B) Blood smears of a patient with iron deficiency anaemia. Note the hypochromic microcytic blood picture with considerable anisopoikilocytosis. Elliptocytes and target cells (asterisks) are found. Thin and elongated elliptocytes are also called pencil cells (arrows).

in circulation. The iron-bound transferrin and TFR complex endocytose to form endosomes. The acidic milieu of the endosomes facilitates release of iron from transferrin and its subsequent transportation into the cytoplasm via DMT1. The apotransferrin (unbound transferrin) undergoes exocytosis, and TFR is recycled to the cell membrane. Cytoplasmic iron is taken up into mitochondria, where it combines with protoporphyrin to form heme. Heme is transported to the cytoplasm where it combines with $\alpha 2\beta 2$ globin chains to form Hb (Figure 34.1A).

34.5 CAUSES

Iron deficiency anaemia (IDA) is the most common cause of anaemia worldwide. In developed countries, IDA in otherwise healthy women at reproductive age is mainly caused by blood loss in the genital tract through menstruation. As blood loss is cumulative, women with apparently normal menstruation could develop IDA. Uterine fibroid is a frequent risk factor associated with heavy menstruation. This is a chronic and continuous process, and patients may not be aware of it until profound anaemia has ensued. In post-menopausal women and in men, IDA is mostly caused by blood loss via the gastrointestinal tract (GIT). In the upper GIT, gastric and duodenal ulcers and gastritis are common causes, for instance, due to *Helicobacter pylori* infection, anti-platelet agents, anti-coagulants or non-steroidal anti-inflammatory drugs. In the lower GIT, colorectal cancers, haemorrhoids and angiodysplasia are frequent causes. Contribution of dietary iron to the total iron store is minimal, except in circumstances where absorption is chronically impaired because of gastrectomy and surgical bypass of the duodenum. Insufficient dietary intake of iron is extremely rare in developed countries, except in anorexia nervosa. IDA due to blood loss through the urinary tract is also extremely rare. An exception is paroxysmal nocturnal haemoglobinuria (PNH) that causes chronic intravascular haemolysis because of defective complement regulation.

34.6 SYMPTOMS

Patients with IDA may present with symptomatic anaemia, including malaise, reduced exercise tolerance, palpitation and shortness of breath particularly on exertion. Patients may also present with symptoms of the clinical conditions that give rise to blood loss, including menorrhagia, epigastric discomfort, passage of tarry stool or rectal bleeding. Prolonged and severe IDA may give rise to painless glossitis, angular stomatitis and brittle or spoon-shaped nails, known as koilonychia.

34.7 INVESTIGATIONS

Investigations are usually initiated by the presence of hypochromic microcytic anaemia, with or without reactive thrombocytosis (Figure 34.1B). A review of blood film is essential and is characterised by the presence of hypochromic and microcytic cells, variable red cell size and shape, known as anisopoikilocytosis, elliptocytes and target cells. Thin and elongated elliptocytes are also called pencil cells. Diagnosis of IDA is ascertained biochemically by a low serum iron and raised total iron–binding capacity (TIBC). TIBC correlates with the total transferrin level whose synthesis in the liver is increased upon iron depletion. Serum transferrin saturation, which is derived by the division of serum iron by TIBC, is typically low. Although a low ferritin level is classically associated with IDA, it is an acute phase reactant and can be released from the liver in case of liver injury. Therefore, its level can be raised in inflammatory or liver disease, and a normal ferritin level does not rule out IDA.

The main differential diagnoses of hypochromic microcytic anaemia in adult patients include previously undiagnosed thalassaemia minor or trait and occasionally, anaemia due to chronic diseases with a hypochromic and microcytic blood picture. For thalassaemia, family history and previous laboratory results from the patient are important. For anaemia due to chronic diseases, a reduced level of TIBC in the relevant clinical context distinguishes itself from IDA. Anaemia in both situations is usually modest, unlike IDA, in which the extent of anaemia can be profound.

Once a diagnosis of IDA has been made, the underlying causes should be identified. In men or in post-menopausal women, upper and/or lower endoscopy should be performed to identify possible blood loss through the GIT. In women at reproductive age, without any GI symptoms, a gynaecological assessment including pelvic ultrasound should be performed to identify uterine fibroid.

Rarely, haematological investigations for PNH may be needed for patients with intermittent dark coloured urine.

34.8 TREATMENT

Oral iron supplement is the mainstay for IDA. Ferrous sulfate is the most frequently used preparation, which is given in divided doses on an empty stomach. In general, it takes about 3–6 months of supplement to replenish the iron store. In patients for whom a more rapid increase in haemoglobin is desirable or oral supplement has not been effective, iron can be replenished via the parenteral route. One single dose may suffice to replenish the depleted iron store in the body, and Hb usually responds in 1–2 weeks. At present, two preparations of parenteral iron supplement are available, namely, ferric carboxymaltose and iron isomaltoside.

34.9 KEY POINTS

1. Diagnosis of IDA should prompt investigations for underlying blood loss from the body.
2. Hepcidin is the key hormone regulating iron metabolism. It blocks iron transport in the macrophages and intestinal epithelial cells.
3. Both oral and intravenous iron supplements are available. The latter gives a more rapid response in Hb.

ADDITIONAL READINGS

1. Camaschella C. Iron deficiency anemia. New Engl J Med 2015; 372: 19.
2. Andrews NC. Disorders of iron metabolism. New Engl J Med 1999; 341: 1986–1995.

35 Vitamin B12 Deficiency Anaemia

35.1 CLINICAL SCENARIO

A 64-year-old man with well-controlled hypertension and diabetes presented with exertional shortness of breath and fatigue for the past 2 weeks. In fact, he had an episode of non-syncopal fall a few days before but had not sought medical advice. Except for profound pallor and mild ankle oedema, physical examination was unremarkable.

35.2 LABORATORY REPORTS

	Results	Reference Range	Units
Haemoglobin	3.2	11.5–14.8	g/dL
Mean corpuscular volume	124	82.0–95.5	fL
White cell count	1.92	3.89–9.93	10^9/L
Platelet count	47	167–396	10^9/L
Reticulocyte count	1.52	0.8–2.51	%
Lactate dehydrogenase	3270	118–221	IU/L
Total bilirubin	50	4–23	μmol/L

Blood film showed anisopoikilocytosis, macrocytosis, a few schistocytes, hypersegmented neutrophils and macro-ovalocytes (Figure 35.1A).

35.3 QUESTIONS

1. What are the haematologic abnormalities?
2. What are the potential causes?
3. What is the treatment approach?

35.4 CLINICAL PROGRESS

The constellations of laboratory abnormalities including macrocytic anaemia, pancytopenia, biochemical evidence of haemolysis and characteristic hypersegmented neutrophils and macro-ovalocytes suggested the diagnosis of vitamin B12 deficiency anaemia.

35.5 FURTHER LABORATORY TESTS

	Results	Reference Range	Units
Serum holotranscobalamin	< 5	> 46.2	pmol/L
RBC folate	9.9	3.2–19.8	μg/L
Anti-parietal cell antibody	Positive	Negative	
Anti-intrinsic factor antibody	> 200	< 20	RU/mL

DOI: 10.1201/9781003325413-41

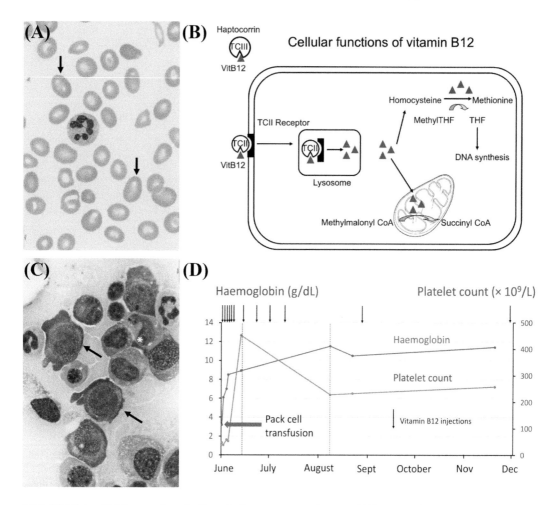

FIGURE 35.1 (A) Macrocytic red cells and a hypersegmented neutrophil in megaloblastic anaemia (Wright-Giemsa × 1000). Macro-ovalocytes were encountered (arrows). (B) Cellular function of Vitamin B12. TC: Transcobalamin; THF: Tetrahydrofolate. (C) Megaloblasts (arrows) and a giant band cell (asterisk) in megaloblastic anaemia (Wright-Giemsa × 1000). Bone marrow examination is not routinely performed in Vitamin B12 deficiency anaemia. (D) Haematological responses to vitamin B12 replacement.

Upper endoscopy showed atrophic gastritis. Biopsy showed no evidence of *Helicobacter pylori* infection or malignancy.

35.6   SOURCES OF VITAMIN B12 IN THE BODY

Vitamin B12 is naturally synthesised by micro-organisms, and our body store of vitamin B12 is dependent on dietary intake. In herbivorous animals, the gastrointestinal tract supports the growth of micro-organisms that synthesise vitamin B12, which is subsequently absorbed and incorporated into body tissues. In humans, vitamin B12 is generally acquired from animal tissues or dairy products including milk, cheese and eggs. Vitamin B12 can also be acquired in fortified cereals or nutritional yeasts, fermented soybeans and vitamin supplements. In the large intestine and caecum, bacterial synthesis of vitamin B12 may take place, but it cannot be absorbed and readily utilised.

35.7 DIETARY VITAMIN B12 ABSORPTION

Dietary vitamin B12 is released in the stomach by gastric acid and the digestion of food by pepcin. Haptocorrin (HC) secreted by salivary glands binds vitamin B12 in the stomach. When the gastric content enters the duodenum, HC becomes digested by the pancreatic proteases in an alkaline environment, and vitamin B12 becomes attached to intrinsic factor (IF) that is secreted by the gastric parietal cells. The vitamin B12–IF complex binds to specific receptors in the terminal ileum, where it is endocytosed. IF is degraded by lysosomal proteases, and vitamin B12 is exported to the circulation by an ATP-driven exporter, multidrug resistance protein (MRP), where it binds to transcobalamin (TC) or HC. TC is ubiquitously synthesised and circulated in predominantly unsaturated form, with only about 10% of TC normally being bound to vitamin B12. When TC carries vitamin B12, it is known as both holotranscobalamin (holoTC) and active fraction vitamin B12 as it is taken up by cells, where vitamin B12 performs its physiologic function. HC is almost fully saturated with vitamin B12, and evidence of cellular uptake of vitamin B12 bound to HC is scarce. It generally takes 1–2 years to deplete the body's store of vitamin B12 in patients whose absorption is perturbed by, for instance, gastrectomy or terminal ileum resection.

35.8 CELLULAR FUNCTION OF VITAMIN B12

Vitamin B12 is needed for most body tissues, and it serves as a cofactor for two enzymes, *viz.*, methionine synthase and l-methylmalonyl–coenzyme A (CoA) mutase in two cellular processes: DNA synthesis and intermediary metabolism. Following receptor-mediated endocytosis of holoTC, the holoTC-receptor complex is degraded in lysosomes, and vitamin B12 is released into the cytoplasm, where it is required by methionine synthase (MS) in the cytosol and methylmalonyl-CoA mutase (MCM) in the mitochondria as methylcobalamin and adenosylcobalamin. Methylcobalamin is essential for the remethylation of homocysteine to methionine by MS. In this process, 5-methyltetrahydrofolate (5-MTHF) supplies the methyl group and is converted to tetrahydrofolate. Methionine is subsequently adenosylated to S-adenosylmethionine (SAM) to supply methyl groups that are critical for the methylation of proteins, phospholipids, neurotransmitters, RNA, and DNA. In contrast, adenosylcobalamin is a cofactor for MCM, and it catalyses the conversion of methylmalonyl-CoA to succinyl-CoA. As methylmalonyl-CoA is a degradation product of propionate, this reaction serves to degrade odd-chain fatty acids and certain amino acids and cholesterol and supply their metabolites to the tricarboxylic acid cycle (Figure 35.1B).

35.9 CLINICAL MANIFESTATIONS

Subclinical vitamin B12 deficiency is thought to precede the onset of full-blown features of vitamin B12 deficiency anaemia. Symptoms may be absent or non-specific, and a high index of suspicion is needed. Typically, signs and symptoms of vitamin B12 deficiency include those of **anaemia**, e.g., malaise, exertional dyspnoea, palpitation and dizziness; **neurological defects**, e.g., numbness and tingling sensations in extremities, muscle weakness and unsteady gait; **neuropsychiatric defects**, e.g., depression and psychosis; **gastrointestinal symptoms**, e.g., sore tongue and mouth and epigastric discomfort; and **autoimmunity**, e.g., early graying of hairs, alopecia, brittle nails.

35.10 LABORATORY FEATURES

Clinical suspicion and work up for vitamin B12 deficiency anaemia usually begins with the findings of macrocytic anaemia. Mean corpuscular volume (MCV) can be as high as > 120 fL, which is uncommon in other causes of macrocytosis. In severe cases, leukopenia and thrombocytopenia may occur. Typical blood film shows macrocytosis, macro-ovalocytes and neutrophil hypersegmentation;

this is defined by the presence of any neutrophils with more than 5 nuclear segments (lobes) or at least 5% of neutrophils with 5 nuclear segments (rule of 5). Biochemically, raised lactate dehydrogenase (LDH) and unconjugated hyperbilirubinaemia are commonly seen, reflecting haemolysis of megaloblasts in the bone marrow, i.e., intramedullary haemolysis due to ineffective haematopoiesis. In contrast to other causes of haemolysis, profound polychromasia, spherocytosis or schistocytes are absent. Serum vitamin B12 assay used to be the standard practice for the diagnosis of vitamin B12 deficiency. It measures the circulatory concentration of vitamin B12 bound to both holoTC (active form) and HC (inactive form). More recently, the serum holoTC level has been used to evaluate the bioactive vitamin B12 status and is predicated on the idea that it is biologically more relevant and has significantly higher diagnostic sensitivity. Increases in total plasma homocysteine and methylmalonic acid are sensitive markers of vitamin B12 deficiency at the tissue level, and a rapid decrease of these levels upon vitamin B12 supplement could be useful for the diagnosis of vitamin B12 deficiency anaemia. However, these tests are not widely available in the laboratory, which limits their clinical applications.

35.11   BONE MARROW FEATURES

Bone marrow examination is usually not required for the diagnosis of vitamin B12 deficiency anaemia, except in circumstances where clinical and laboratory findings are inconsistent with the diagnosis or patients do not respond to vitamin B12 supplement. An important differential diagnosis is myelodysplastic syndrome. The typical bone marrow features of vitamin B12 deficiency are those of megaloblastic anaemia, which is characterised functionally by ineffective erythropoiesis and morphologically by the presence of megaloblasts, i.e., late erythroid precursors with an immature nucleus and relatively mature cytoplasm (nuclear–cytoplasmic asynchrony) due to impaired DNA synthesis. Myelopoiesis is also affected and is characterised by the presence of giant metamyelocytes and band cells. The megakaryocytes are also large and hyperlobulated (Figure 35.1C).

35.12   CAUSES

Although a low serum level of vitamin B12 may be seen in different conditions, including people on vegetarian or vegan diets, people on long-term metformin or proton pump inhibitors or individuals who are pregnant or ageing, a full-blown picture of vitamin B12 deficiency anaemia is encountered in only a few clinical settings. The body store of vitamin B12 is generally sufficient for 1–2 years in the absence of dietary intake. Patients undergoing gastrectomy, gastric bypass surgery or terminal ileum resection should receive parenteral vitamin B12 replacement; otherwise, they may develop vitamin B12 deficiency anaemia 1–2 years afterwards. In patients without a surgical history, the most common cause of vitamin B12 deficiency anaemia is pernicious anaemia. Other causes are generally rare.[1]

35.13   PERNICIOUS ANAEMIA

Pernicious anaemia (PA) is an autoimmune gastritis resulting from the destruction of gastric parietal cells, hence the lack of intrinsic factor to bind ingested vitamin B12. The immune response is directed against the gastric H/K–ATPase, leading to achlorhydria. As an autoimmune disorder, PA is associated with thyroid disease, type 1 diabetes mellitus, vitiligo and early greying of hair. The median age of onset is about 60–70 years old with a slight female preponderance. The diagnosis of PA begins with the aforementioned clinical and haematological features of vitamin B12 deficiency and clinical features of autoimmunity. Once biochemical evidence of vitamin B12 deficiency can be ascertained, antibodies associated with PA should be tested. Specifically, anti-parietal cell (PC) antibody is associated with high sensitivity but low specificity. In the absence of clinical, haematological and biochemical evidence of vitamin B12 deficiency, a positive anti-PC antibody, even in the presence of anaemia, is of little diagnostic value. Anti-intrinsic factor (IF) antibody is associated with low sensitivity but high specificity. Therefore, a negative anti-IF antibody cannot rule out PA. Upper endoscopy should be performed to confirm gastritis and to rule out adenocarcinoma of stomach. The Schilling test, based on urinary excretion of ingested radioactive vitamin B12 as a surrogate of intestinal absorption, is obsolete in most laboratories.

35.14 TREATMENT

In principle, patients with documented vitamin B12 deficiency anaemia should have rapid replenishment followed by life-long maintenance. Generally, patients should receive intramuscular or subcutaneous injection of vitamin B12 at 1000 µg daily for 1 week, followed by the same dose given weekly for 4 weeks, then once every 1 to 3 months. The daily vitamin B12 injections at the initial phase of treatment will lead to hypokalaemia and hypophosphataemia, and serum electrolytes should be monitored in the first week of treatment. Haematological response is often delayed with an increase in reticulocyte and platelet counts occurring in the first 1–2 weeks and correction of anaemia after 6–8 weeks (Figure 35.1D). Neurological symptoms may respond weeks to months after supplement, depending on the severity and duration of symptoms before replacement. More recently, a daily oral dose of 1000 µg vitamin B12 has been shown to achieve comparable replenishment via diffusion in the mucosal epithelium, even in the context of PA.

35.15 KEY POINTS

1. Vitamin B12 plays an important role in DNA synthesis and intermediary metabolism at the cellular level.
2. Vitamin B12 deficiency anaemia is characterised by distinct clinical, haematological and biochemical features.
3. PA is the most common medical cause of Vitamin B12 deficiency anaemia.

ADDITIONAL READING

1. Stabler SP. Vitamin B12 deficiency. N Engl J Med 2013; 368: 149–160.

Haemolytic Anaemia

36 Warm-Type Autoimmune Haemolytic Anaemia

36.1 CLINICAL SCENARIO

A 73-year-old woman with well-controlled hypertension and diabetes presented with fever and shortness of breath. She was pale, but otherwise, physical examination was unremarkable.

36.2 LABORATORY REPORTS

	Results	References	Units
Haemoglobin	4.0	11.5–14.8	g/dL
Mean corpuscular volume	96.7	82–95.5	fL
White cell count	8.0	3.89–9.93	10^9/L
Platelet count	256	167–396	10^9/L
Reticulocyte count	13	0.5–2.5	%
Lactate dehydrogenase	683	120–220	IU/L
Total bilirubin	67	4–20	μmol/L
Haptoglobin	Undetectable	0.5–2.2	g/L

Blood film showed the presence of spherocytes and polychromasia (Figure 36.1A). Direct anti-globulin test (DAT) was positive (polyspecific and anti-immunoglobulin [Ig] G positive, anti-C3d negative) (Figure 36.1B). Bone marrow showed erythroid hyperplasia with no abnormal infiltration. Flow cytometry of bone marrow aspirate showed no clonal B-cells. Positron emission tomography/Computed tomography (PET/CT) scan showed no abnormal lymphadenopathy. Autoimmune screen, serum protein electrophoresis and cold agglutinin were negative.

36.3 QUESTIONS

1. What is the diagnosis?
2. What are the triggering and underlying factors?
3. What is the management plan?

36.4 DIAGNOSIS

The presence of macrocytic anaemia, raised lactate dehydrogenase (LDH), unconjugated bilirubin and undetectable haptoglobin suggested a haemolytic process. This was supported by the presence of polychromasia and spherocytosis. In this context, a positive DAT confirmed the diagnosis of autoimmune haemolytic anaemia (AIHA). In particular, positive anti-IgG and negative anti-C3d suggested warm-type AIHA. In half of the cases, known as primary AIHA, no underlying cause can be identified. In another half, causative factors can be identified, including drug exposure, notably methyldopa, high-dose penicillin, cephalosporin, purine analogues and immune checkpoint inhibitors, and immunologic or lymphoproliferative disorders and infection, including recent cases of severe acute respiratory syndrome coronavirus 2 (SARS-CoV-2). The lack of drug intake causative of AIHA, negative serum protein electrophoresis, bone marrow examination, PET/CT and autoimmune markers supported the diagnosis of primary AIHA in this patient.

DOI: 10.1201/9781003325413-43

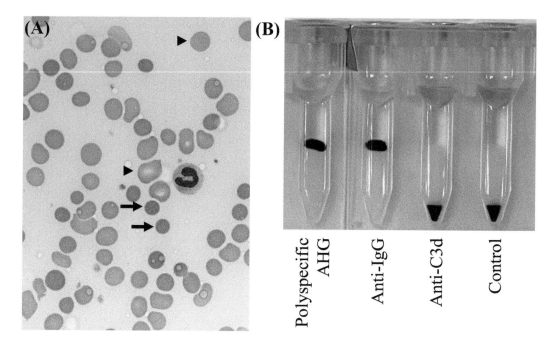

FIGURE 36.1 (A) Peripheral blood smear showing polychromasia and spherocytosis (Wright-Giemsa ×
1000). (B) Direct antiglobulin test (DAT) by solid phase micro-column agglutination method. The anti-human
globulin (AHG) reagents are embedded in the beads of the micro-column. After applying the red cells for testing and centrifugation, sensitised antibody-coated red cells are trapped at the top part of the micro-column,
while negative red cells sink to the bottom. From left to right: Polyspecific AHG (+), anti-IgG (+), anti-C3d
(−) and control (−).

36.5   PATHOGENESIS

Warm-type AIHA is generally defined by the presence of antibodies that show the highest affinity
to antigen at 37°C. The autoantibodies are polyclonal and are produced by nonclonal B lymphocytes
and plasma cells, even in the presence of underlying clonal B-cell lymphoproliferative disease. They
show broad specificities to red cell antigens in contrast to cold autoantibodies that target I/i antigens
or the biphasic Donath–Landsteiner (DL) antibody that targets the P antigen. They are usually IgG,
but rarely, IgM and IgA warm antibodies have been reported. Typically, erythrocytes are opsonised
with IgG and are either directly phagocytosed by splenic macrophages or become spherocytes and
subsequently phagocytosed. In half of the cases, IgG-mediated complement activation occurs, and
the complement fragment 3b (C3b)–coated cells become phagocytosed by hepatic macrophages.
This is evident by the presence of C3d–coated circulating red cells. Rarely, cleavage of C5 and
activation of the terminal complement cascade occur, resulting in the formation of membrane attack
complex and intravascular haemolysis. Furthermore, T-lymphocytes may be involved, specifically
via perturbation of immune checkpoints due to cytotoxic T-lymphocyte antigen 4 (CTLA-4) poly-
morphism or cancer treatment targeting immune checkpoint inhibitors of the programmed cell
death 1 (PD-1) signal pathway.

36.6   DIFFERENTIAL DIAGNOSIS

There are a number of differential diagnoses for patients with anaemia and positive DAT. In fact,
positive DAT can occur in healthy donors or in up to 10% of hospitalised patients unrelated to
AIHA. Therefore, positive DAT should only be interpreted in the context of proven haemolysis;

otherwise, anaemia could be due to other causes, and a positive DAT may lead to misdiagnosis of AIHA. In patients with AIHA and an anti-IgG positive DAT, particularly in children after viral infection, **paroxysmal cold haemoglobinuria** (PCH) should be considered. In PCH, the autoantibody is a biphasic IgG haemolysin known as Donath–Lansteiner antibody. It binds to red cell antigen at temperatures below central body temperature but activates the terminal complement cascade after warming to 37°C in the core, resulting in intravascular haemolysis. Another differential diagnosis is **mixed warm and cold AIHA**, defined by the presence of warm IgG autoantibody and a high titre of cold agglutinins. Clinical course is often more severe, response to treatment is less satisfactory and prognosis is worse than warm AIHA. However, up to 10% of AIHA can occur in patients whose **DAT is negative**. This can be due to the low density of immunoglobulin, complement or both on red cells or rarely, due to IgA AIHA as most polyspecific reagents do not include anti-IgA. Non-immune causes of haemolysis should always be ruled out.

36.7 MANAGEMENT

Primary warm-type AIHA should be treated with corticosteroid as the first line of treatment. About 80% of patients will respond, and steroids should be tapered over a few months. Patients who relapse or are steroid refractory should receive anti-CD20 antibody rituximab with a response rate of up to 80%. Splenectomy should be offered to patients who relapse or who are refractory to rituximab with a response rate of nearly 70%. Other salvage treatment includes alternative immunosuppressive agents and bortezomib. Folic acid supplement should be given. Blood transfusion in warm-type AIHA patients is challenging due to the presence of autoantibodies that interfere with red cell typing and antibody screen. Extended cell phenotype before transfusion should be performed, and phenotype-matched red cells can be given despite the presence of interfering antibodies. A number of targeted therapies are being evaluated for the treatment of warm-type AIHA, notably, agents that target T-cells (e.g., alemtuzumab), B-cells (e.g., ibrutinib, venetoclax and idelalisib) and plasma cells (e.g., daratumumab), agents that complement C1q and C3 inhibitors and spleen tyrosine kinase inhibitor fostamatinib that perturbs red cell phagocytosis.

36.8 KEY POINTS

1. Positive DAT should be interpreted in the context of established haemolytic anaemia.
2. AIHA can be primary or secondary to causative factors.
3. In warm-type AIHA, the autoantibodies are polyclonal and mostly IgG and show broad specificities.
4. Corticosteroid is the first line of treatment. Steroid refractory cases should be treated by rituximab.

ADDITIONAL READINGS

1. Berentsen S, Barcellini W. Autoimmune hemolytic anemias. N Engl J Med 2021; 385: 1407–1419.
2. Barcellini W, Fattizzo B. How I treat warm autoimmune hemolytic anemia. Blood 2021; 137(10): 1283–1294.
3. McKnight TF, DiGuardo MA, Jacob EK. New developments in the understanding and treatment of autoimmune hemolytic anemia: traditional and novel tests. Hematol Oncol Clin N Am 2022; 36: 293–305.
4. Kuter DJ. Warm autoimmune hemolytic anemia and the best treatment strategies. Hematology Am Soc Hematol Educ Program 2022 Dec 9; 2022(1): 105–113.

37 Cold Agglutinin Disease

37.1 CLINICAL SCENARIO

A 90-year-old-man presented with purplish colouration of the fingertips, toes and nose tip in cold weather for 6 years. He had retroperitoneal leiomyosarcoma with surgical excision 20 years ago and gout and hypertension on amlodipine and irbesartan. He had the thalassaemia trait, and his elder sister died of liver cancer. His usual haemoglobin was about 9 g/dL.

37.2 LABORATORY REPORTS

	Results	Reference	Units
Haemoglobin	6.4	13–17	g/dL
White cell count	8	4–10	10^9/L
Platelet count	285	154–371	10^9/L
Reticulocyte count	2.0	0.5–2.0	%
Lactate dehydrogenase	496	120–220	IU/L
Total bilirubin	28	4–20	μmol/L
Immunoglobulin (Ig) M	568	55–300	mg/dL
Paraprotein IgM/κ	4.79	Absent	g/L

Blood smear showed that red cell agglutination and cold agglutinin titre against normal adult (I+) cells at 4°C was greater than 8192.

Direct antiglobulin test:	Positive
Anti-human globulin (polyspecific):	Positive
Anti-immunoglobulin G:	Weakly positive
Anti-complement (anti-C3d):	Positive

37.3 QUESTIONS

1. What is the likely diagnosis?
2. What could be the underlying causes?
3. What is the treatment of choice?

37.4 CLINICAL PROGRESS

The patient's bone marrow showed no evidence of lymphoma involvement. Positron emission tomography/Computed tomography (PET/CT) scan also showed no lymphadenopathy or organomegaly. A diagnosis of cold agglutinin disease was made. He was given 4 weekly doses of rituximab and a regular folic acid supplement. His haemoglobin dropped during wintertime, consistent with the cold-induced haemolytic anaemia (Figure 37.1A).

37.5 COLD AGGLUTININ DISEASE

Cold agglutinin disease (CAD) is defined as autoimmune haemolytic anaemia (AIHA) where the autoantibody is a cold agglutinin, and apparently no underlying clinical disease can be identified.

DOI: 10.1201/9781003325413-44

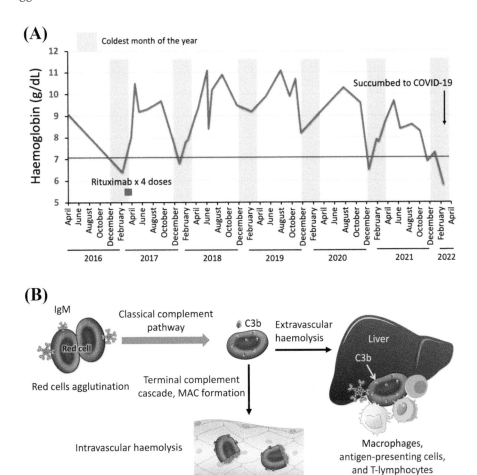

FIGURE 37.1 (A) Seasonal variation of haemoglobin levels in a cold agglutinin disease (CAD) patient, reflecting the effects of ambient temperature on disease activity. (B) Pathogenesis of CAD.

Cold agglutinin (CA) refers to autoantibodies mostly monoclonal immunoglobulin (Ig) M/κ with anti-I specificity, that bind to antigen at 0–4°C and agglutinate red cells. Some CA can agglutinate red cells at a much higher temperature, e.g., ≥ 28°C. When our fingers, toes, nose or ears are exposed to cold, their local temperature can be as low as 28°C, and these CA become pathological. CAD accounts for up to one-third of AIHA. Technically, CAD is defined as autoimmune haemolytic disease with a direct antiglobulin test strongly positive for C3d and negative or only weakly positive for IgG and a CA titre of > 64 at 4°C. The definition was based on previous observations that innocuous CA may be present in the general population and that they are polyclonal and in titre < 64.

37.6   PATHOGENESIS OF HAEMOLYSIS IN CAD

As blood circulates to the acral parts that are exposed to cold, monoclonal IgM CA bind the red cell surface and activate the classical complement pathway via C1 activation. As the red cells carrying the bound Ig-C1 complex circulate to the warmer core circulation, C1q esterase activates C4 and C2 and generates the C3 convertase. The C3 convertase cleaves C3 into C3a and C3b. Red cells coated with C3b, i.e., opsonised, are sequestered by macrophages in the reticuloendothelial system, particularly Kupffer cells in the liver where they are haemolysed (Figure 37.1B). C3b can be further cleaved into C3c and C3d, and C3d is detectable in a direct antiglobulin test. Occasionally, C3b can bind with C4b and C2b to form C5 convertase that leads to initiation of a terminal complement cascade, culminating in membrane attack complex (MAC) and intravascular haemolysis (Figure 37.1B).

37.7   COLD AGGLUTININ SYNDROME

This is an emerging entity in which the CA-mediated AIHA is secondary to underlying diseases including specific infection (mycoplasma pneumoniae, Epstein–Barr virus, cytomegalovirus and SARS-CoV-2 infection) or underlying lymphoproliferative diseases, typically Waldenström macroglobulinaemia, chronic lymphocytic leukaemia or other low-grade lymphomas.

37.8   INVESTIGATIONS

Patients with cold-type AIHA and CA titre > 64 should have serum protein electrophoresis to look for monoclonal IgM/κ and should be investigated for underlying infective causes and lymphoproliferative diseases based on bone marrow examination and PET/CT scan. Furthermore, hepatitis B serology should be checked especially when patients may receive anti-CD20 therapy. It is important that all blood samples are pre-warmed at 37°C before analysis.

37.9   TREATMENT

Patients with CAD should be advised to avoid cold exposure to their acral parts. Asymptomatic patients with mild anaemia may only need folic acid supplement. Patients with symptomatic anaemia will need transfusion of pre-warmed packed cells, and in addition to a folic acid supplement, they will need specific therapy for CAD. Rarely, patients with severe acrocyanosis and digital gangrene may need prompt clearance of CA, and plasmapheresis should be considered. It is important to know that unlike warm-type AIHA, corticosteroid and splenectomy are of minimal benefit in the management of CAD. Anti-CD20 monoclonal antibody rituximab is the mainstay of treatment with about 50% of patients showing a response. Combination of rituximab with purine analogue fludarabine or bendamustine may increase the response rate to 70% at the expense of increased toxicity due to opportunistic infections. More recently, a complement inhibitor sutimlimab, which selectively inhibits C1s, was shown to reduce transfusion dependence of CAD patients by reducing haemolysis and was approved by the FDA for this indication.

37.10   KEY POINTS

1. CAD is a type of AIHA triggered by exposure to cold. When it is secondary to underlying diseases, including infection and lymphoproliferative diseases, it is known as cold agglutinin syndrome.
2. CA is autoantibody, mostly monoclonal IgM/κ with anti-I specificity, that binds to antigen at 0–4°C and agglutinates red cells. Some CA can agglutinate red cells at a much higher temperature, e.g., ≥ 28°C, causing clinical disease.
3. The mainstay of CAD treatment is avoidance of cold exposure and anti-CD20 monoclonal antibody. Unlike warm-type AIHA, corticosteroid and splenectomy are not effective.

ADDITIONAL READINGS

1. Berentsen S. How I treat cold agglutinin disease. Blood 2021; 137(10): 1295–1303.
2. Berentsen S, Barcellini W. Autoimmune haemolytic anemia. N Engl J Med 2021; 381: 1407–1419.
3. Gabbard AP, Booth GS. Cold agglutinin disease. Clin Haematol Int 2020; 2(3): 95–100.

38 G6PD Deficiency

38.1 CLINICAL SCENARIO

A 66-year-old man with a history of biliary pancreatitis and gallstones presented with a 1-week history of jaundice and tea-coloured urine. He has taken herbal medicine for 2 months as a health remedy and was given a course of nitrofurantoin by his general practitioner for urinary tract infection 1 week ago. At presentation, he was jaundiced, and his temperature was 37.7°C. Physical examination was otherwise unremarkable.

38.2 LABORATORY REPORTS

	Results	References	Units
Haemoglobin	7.4	13.3–17.1	g/dL
Mean corpuscular volume	97.1	82–95.5	fL
White cell count	6.04	3.9–10	10^9/L
Platelet count	255	167–396	10^9/L
Reticulocyte count	3.07	0.8–2.51	%
Lactate dehydrogenase	387	118–221	U/L
Total bilirubin	33	4–23	μmol/L

Blood smear showed the presence of hemighosts, bite cells and polychromasia, suggestive of oxidative haemolysis (Figure 38.1A).

38.3 QUESTIONS

1. What is the main haematological problem?
2. What is the next haematological blood test?
3. What is/are the triggering factor(s) for the patient's condition?

38.4 CLINICAL PROGRESS

Additional laboratory tests were as follows:

	Results	References	Units
Fluorescent spot	Abnormal	Normal	
G6PD assay	4	6.35–10.33	IU/g Hb

38.5 G6PD PHYSIOLOGY

Glucose-6-phosphate dehydrogenase (G6PD) is an evolutionarily conserved enzyme that catalyses the rate-limiting step of the pentose phosphate pathway (PPP), which converts glucose-6-phosphate to 6-phosphoglucono-δ-lactone. The PPP produces pentose sugar that is required for nucleic acid synthesis. In addition, nicotinamide adenine dinucleotide phosphate (NADP) is converted to its reduced form, NADPH, during the process (Figure 38.1B). NADPH converts glutathione disulfide

DOI: 10.1201/9781003325413-45

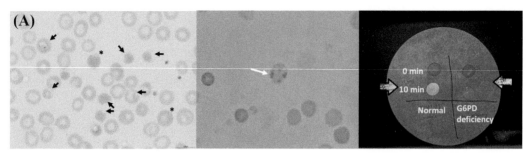

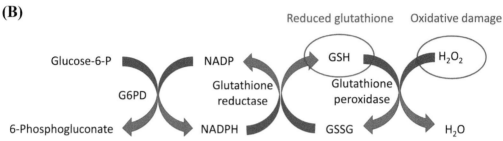

FIGURE 38.1 (A) Left panel: Blood film showing the presence of "hemighosts" and "bite cells" (arrows), basophilic stippling (arrow) and polychromasia (asterisks) in acute glucose-6-phosphate dehydrogenase (G6PD) haemolysis (Wright-Giemsa × 1000). Middle panel: Heinz bodies (arrow) in oxidative haemolysis (supravital stain × 1000). Right panel: Fluorescent spot test. A small amount of blood was incubated with glucose-6-phosphate and nicotinamide adenine dinucleotide phosphate (NADP) in the substrate reagent and spotted on filter paper. Once dried, the spots were viewed under long-wave ultraviolet (UV) light—the by-product of the reaction (NADPH) is fluorescent. NADPH fluorescence is directly proportional to G6PD activity, and a lack of fluorescence indicates G6PD deficiency. At time zero, no fluorescence was detected. After incubation at 37°C for 10 minutes, the normal sample on the left showed detectable fluorescence under UV light, while the sample on the right showed G6PD deficiency. (B) Molecular pathways of G6PD leading to the protection of red cells from oxidative damage. G6PD: Glucose-6-P: Glucose-6-Phosphate; GSH: Reduced glutathione; GSSG: Glutathione disulfide; H_2O_2: Hydrogen peroxide.

(GSSG) to reduced glutathione (GSH), which is the scavenger of free radicals and prevents cellular damage from reactive oxygen species (ROS). Furthermore, NADPH is the electron donor required for the biosynthesis of DNA, fatty acids and steroids and is the coenzyme of cytochrome P450 required for the metabolism of drugs and xenobiotics. G6PD is a ubiquitous enzyme, but red blood cells (RBC) are particularly dependent on it because i) mature RBC cannot generate proteins are hence particularly vulnerable to their oxidation, ii) the G6PD/NADPH pathway is the only source of GSH in RBC and iii) RBC are subject to endogenous oxidative stress because of the high intra-cellular concentration of haemoglobin that binds oxygen. Under physiological conditions, G6PD activity decreases from a high level in reticulocytes to only one-tenth of this level in senescent RBC. In G6PD-deficient RBC, reticulocytes show lower-than-normal G6PD activity that undergoes rapid and exponential decay as they differentiate into mature RBC, and the oldest cells are devoid of G6PD activity, making them vulnerable to oxidative haemolysis.

38.6 GENETICS

G6PD deficiency is a polymorphic genetic trait with more than 230 variants in the coding sequence that are mostly missense mutations or small in-frame deletions, resulting in reduced G6PD activity. Complete absence of G6PD is embryonic lethal. Some of these variants are more prevalent in Asia, Africa and Mediterranean regions, where malaria is endemic, whereas other variants show a worldwide distribution. The G6PD gene is located at the long arm of the X chromosome. Males have only one G6PD allele and can be either normal or hemizygous for G6PD deficiency. Females have two G6PD alleles and can be normal, heterozygous or homozygous for G6PD deficiency, and the latter may occur if their fathers are hemizygous and mothers are heterozygous for G6PD deficiency. Moreover, as the X chromosome undergoes random inactivation (lyonisation), heterozygous females are mosaics for G6PD with a mixture of G6PD normal (defective allele inactivated) and G6PD-deficient (wildtype allele inactivated) RBC. As patients become older, clonal haematopoiesis occurs resulting in skewed lyonisation, i.e., some clones expand at the expense of others. Expansion of a G6PD-deficient clone results in reduced G6PD activity overall.

38.7   HAEMATOLOGICAL EFFECTS

G6PD deficiency is a classic example of pharmacogenetics. Genotypic carriers show no clinical abnormality under physiological conditions. Exposure to certain drugs (Table 38.1), for instance, nitrofurantoin in this patient, and fava bean generates hydrogen peroxide and ROS and in the absence of NADPH due to G6PD deficiency, would have important consequences in RBC. Particularly when GSH in RBC becomes exhausted, the sulfhydryl group of cytoplasmic and membrane proteins become oxidised, causing aggregation and cross-linking in the cell membrane and pathognomonic hemighost under microscopy. Partially denatured haemoglobin binds to membrane cytoskeleton, forming Heinz bodies. RBC with severe damage will undergo intravascular haemolysis. In the surviving RBC, clusters of oxidised band 3 in the membrane bind to immunoglobulin G and complement C3c, resulting in opsonisation and phagocytosis and, thus, extravascular haemolysis.

38.8   DIAGNOSIS

The first clue to the diagnosis is acute non-immune haemolysis, particularly in patients of Asian, African or Mediterranean ethnicity who have been exposed to food or drugs known to cause oxidative damage, specifically when there is a positive family history. There should be biochemical evidence of haemolysis including raised unconjugated bilirubin and lactate dehydrogenase. Haptoglobin is reduced. Haemoglobinuria may occur in severe cases. The pathognomonic haematological feature is the presence of "bite cells" or "hemighosts" (Figure 38.1A). Heinz bodies in RBC, as shown by supravital staining using methyl violet, are indicative of denatured haemoglobin. Polychromasia is characteristic. Direct antiglobulin test should be performed, and a negative result helps rule out immune-mediated haemolysis. The screening for G6PD deficiency is by Beutler fluorescent spot test, a rapid and inexpensive test that detects NADPH produced by G6PD under ultraviolet light. Absence of fluorescence is indicative of G6PD deficiency (Figure 38.1A). Quantitative assay for G6PD activity should also be performed. False negative results may occur after transfusion or during active haemolysis as reticulocytes may show higher G6PD activity.

TABLE 38.1

Examples of Drugs Associated with Oxidative Haemolysis in G6PD Deficiency

Dapsone
Primaquine
Ciprofloxacin, moxifloxacin, ofloxacin
Nitrofurantoin
Rasburicase
Sulfamethoxazole/cotrimoxazole

38.9   MANAGEMENT

Prompt diagnosis is critical, and the inciting agents should be avoided. Mild cases can be managed conservatively with hydration and symptomatic treatment. Patients with severe haemolysis should be managed with transfusion, and those with acute kidney injury due to intravascular haemolysis and haemoglobinaemia should be managed with exchange transfusion and haemodialysis. Family studies are important so that inciting agents can be avoided for otherwise asymptomatic carriers.

38.10   KEY POINTS

1. G6PD deficiency presents with acute non-immune haemolysis upon exposure to oxidising agents with red cells showing characteristic features of oxidative damage.
2. G6PD deficiency occurs in both male and female patients.
3. Rapid screening of G6PD deficiency by fluorescent spot test is available.

ADDITIONAL READINGS

1. Luzzatto L, Ally M, Notaro R. Glucose-6-phosphate dehydrogenase deficiency. Blood 2020; 136(11): 1225–1240.
2. Luzzatto L, Arese P. Favism and glucose-6-phosphate dehydrogenase deficiency. New Engl J Med 2018; 378: 60–71.

39 Hereditary Spherocytosis

39.1 CLINICAL SCENARIO

A 30-year-old woman presented with vomiting and diarrhoea for two days, after eating raw fish and salad, and was admitted to hospital for malaise. She had cholecystectomy for gallstones at age 21 years. She was pale with a tinge of jaundice and had a palpable spleen three fingerbreadths below the costal margin. She had no sibling. Her mother had gallstones and cholecystectomy at age 30 years.

39.2 LABORATORY REPORTS

	Results	References	Units
Haemoglobin	6.7	11–14	g/dL
Mean corpuscular volume	94.9	80–95	fL
White cell count	13.36	4–10	10^9/L
Platelet count	127	170–400	10^9/L
Neutrophil count	11.67	2–7	10^9/L
Reticulocyte count	18.51	1–2	%
Total bilirubin	91	4–20	μmol/L
Lactate dehydrogenase	250	100–200	IU/L
Haptoglobin	Undetectable	0.5–2.2	g/L

Blood smears showed the presence of spherocytosis and polychromasia (Figure 39.1A). The mean channel fluorescence (MCF) ratio of eosin-5-maleimide (EMA) staining on red cells was 0.7 (Reference: 0.92–1.08).

39.3 QUESTIONS

1. What is the diagnosis?
2. What is the principle of management?
3. What are the potential complications of this condition?

39.4 HEREDITARY SPHEROCYTOSIS

The likely diagnosis was hereditary spherocytosis (HS). HS is an inherited haemolytic disease occurring in 1 in 2500 of the population and is more common in Caucasians than in Asians. It is inherited as an autosomal dominant (75% of cases) or autosomal recessive (25% of cases) disease. Patients can be asymptomatic or may develop variable degrees of haemolysis. Haemolysis can occur in hitherto asymptomatic patients during intercurrent illnesses including viral infections or during changes in the physiological state such as pregnancy or strenuous exercise. Chronic haemolytic state is associated with anaemia, jaundice, splenomegaly, cholelithiasis and thrombosis. A family history of cholelithiasis often suggests inherited haemolytic disease.

DOI: 10.1201/9781003325413-46

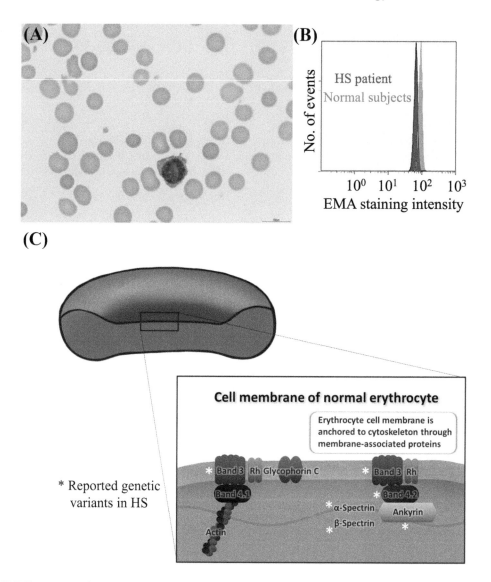

FIGURE 39.1 (A) Spherocytosis and polychromasia in hereditary spherocytosis (HS) (Wright-Giemsa ×
1000). (B) Flow cytometry based on eosin-5-maleimide (EMA) dye showing reduced staining in a hereditary
spherocytosis patient. (C) Red cell membrane proteins and mutation variants in HS (asterisks). Rh: Rhesus
protein.

39.5 DIAGNOSIS

Differential diagnoses of HS include thalassaemia, glucose-6-phosphate dehydrogenase (G6PD)
deficiency and autoimmune haemolytic anaemia (AIHA). In most cases, a detailed family history and peripheral blood smear showing profound spherocytosis suggest the diagnosis of HS.
Previously, osmotic fragility test and acidified glycerol lysis test were standard diagnostic tests.
More recently, eosin-5-maleimide (EMA) binding test is considered more specific for HS and is
less labour-intensive. EMA binds covalently to the plasma membrane proteins of red blood cells
(RBC), including band 3 and other proteins. The mean fluorescence of EMA-stained RBC in HS, as
enumerated by flow cytometry (Figure 39.1B), is lower than the control RBC due to the decreased
amount of target proteins.

39.6   GENETIC BASIS

HS is caused by defective functions of genes that are expressed in the erythrocyte membrane and cytoskeleton. Five genetic variants have been identified, including ankyrin 1 (*ANK1*), spectrin beta, erythrocytic (*SPTB*), solute carrier family 4, member 1 (*SLC4A1*), spectrin alpha, erythrocytic 1 (*SPTA1*) and erythrocyte membrane protein band 4.2 (*EPB42*), which encode the proteins ankyrin, β-spectrin, band 3, α-spectrin and protein 4.2, respectively (Figure 39.1C). Inheritance of variants of *ANK1*, *SPTB*, and *SLC4A1* are autosomal dominant, while *SPTA1* and *EPB42* defects are autosomal recessive. Somatic mutations of these genes have also been reported. Variants of *ANK1* and *SPTB* account for the majority of HS in North America and Europe, whereas those of *EPB42* and *SLC4A1* may be more common in Asia. Defective function of these genes is associated with a decrease in membrane deformability, hence haemolytic anaemia, as RBC transit in the splenic circulation.

39.7   MANAGEMENT

Different genetic variants in HS can give rise to heterogenous clinical manifestations. Patients with mild HS and compensated haemolysis need monitoring and patient education, and immediate medical attendance should be sought in the event of intercurrent illnesses including viral infection, which may precipitate aplastic crises; attention should also be given with respect to symptoms of cholelithiasis and splenomegaly. In patients with profound and prolonged haemolytic anaemia who require repeated transfusions, total or partial splenectomy may be considered. Splenectomy is particularly relevant in paediatric patients, who may be more susceptible to infection post-splenectomy. Alternative causes of haemolytic anaemia should always be considered in the differential diagnoses of patients with established HS.

39.8   KEY POINTS

1. The diagnosis of HS is suggested by a family history of chronic haemolysis and cholelithiasis and profound spherocytosis.
2. Reduced binding of EMA dye to the red cell membrane is considered diagnostic for HS.
3. Five genetic variants are known in HS, and those of *EPB42* and *SLC4A1*, encoding for Protein 4.2 and Band 3 protein, are more common in Asia.

ADDITIONAL READINGS

1. Yang L, Shu H, Zhou M, Gong Y. Literature review on genotype-phenotype correlation in patients with hereditary spherocytosis. Clin Genet 2022; 102(6): 474–482.
2. Kalfa TA. Diagnosis and clinical management of red cell membrane disorders. Hematology Am Soc Hematol Educ Program 2021; 2021(1): 331–340.

40 Paravalvular Leak

40.1 CLINICAL SCENARIO

A 71-year-old-man with chronic rheumatic heart disease and severe mitral stenosis had mechanical mitral and aortic valve replacement in January 2015. He also has had rheumatoid arthritis and interstitial lung disease since 2013. He complained of worsening shortness of breath on exertion in the past 6 months. Transthoracic echocardiogram showed severely dilated left atrium but otherwise normal ejection fraction and prosthesis function. His baseline haemoglobin had been 12–13 g/dL but has become 9–10 g/dL since 1 year before this presentation.

40.2 LABORATORY REPORTS

	Results	References	Units
Haemoglobin	6.8	13.3–17.1	g/dL
Mean corpuscular volume	106.4	82.0–95.5	fL
White cell count	4.6	3.89–9.92	10^9/L
Platelet count	188	154–371	10^9/L
Total bilirubin	52	4–23	μmol/L
Lactate dehydrogenase	2436	118–221	U/L
Serum creatinine	92	67–109	μmol/L

Blood smear: Normal white cell differentials and morphology. Occasional red cell fragments. Polychromasia present (Figure 40.1).

40.3 QUESTIONS

1. What is the haematological abnormality?
2. What is the potential cause and how to confirm it?
3. What is the management plan?

40.4 CLINICAL PROGRESS

The presence of macrocytic anaemia and biochemical evidence of haemolysis would suggest vitamin B12 deficiency with intramedullary haemolysis or haemolytic anaemia. However, the absence of characteristic hypersegmented neutrophils or macro-ovalocytes and the presence of polychromasia were against vitamin B12 deficiency. In fact, the serum level of vitamin B12 was within the normal range. To ascertain the cause of haemolysis, a direct antiglobulin test was performed and was confirmed negative, suggesting that the haemolytic process was non-immune in nature. Urine haemosiderin was positive, and plasma-free haemoglobin was raised, consistent with chronic intravascular haemolysis. A rare but notable cause is paroxysmal nocturnal haemoglobinuria (PNH) due to an acquired *PIG-A* mutation of haematopoietic stem cells. This was ruled out by a negative PNH screening using flow cytometry. As a result, despite apparently normal valvular prosthesis function based on transthoracic echocardiogram, haemolytic anaemia due to a paravalvular leak remains the most likely cause of the patient's anaemia. This was subsequently confirmed by transoesophageal echocardiogram.

DOI: 10.1201/9781003325413-47

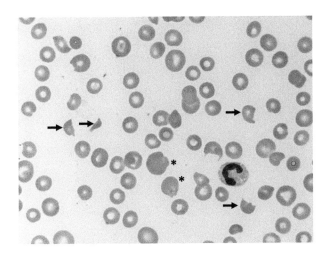

FIGURE 40.1   Microangiopathic change in mechanical haemolytic anaemia showing the presence of schistocytes (arrows) and polychromasia (asterisks) (Wright-Giemsa × 1000).

40.5   CARDIAC PROSTHESIS-RELATED HAEMOLYTIC ANAEMIA

This case illustrates cardiac prosthesis-related haemolytic anaemia, which was first described in the 1950s. With improved prosthesis design and surgical skills, it has become less frequently seen, until more recently when mechanical circulatory support devices and transcatheter valvular interventions became more popular. It is usually diagnosed in the presence of a cardiac prosthesis or mechanical circulatory support device with i) hitherto unexplained and progressive anaemia; ii) red cell destruction with the presence of schistocytes, raised lactate dehydrogenase, unconjugated bilirubin and decreased haptoglobin; and iii) a negative direct antiglobulin test. Transoesophageal rather than transthoracic echocardiogram is often needed to delineate the anatomical defects.

Mechanical valve replacement remains to be the most common cause of cardiac prosthesis-related haemolytic anaemia, and its occurrence has increased with the age of prosthetic valves. It is mostly due to paravalvular leak arising from suture dehiscence due to heavy annular calcification. It also happens in open mitral valve repair and annular ring replacement surgeries due to ring dehiscence, protrusion of paravalvular suture materials, residual free-floating chordae or turbulent eccentric residual regurgitation jets. Furthermore, haemolytic anaemia can occur after transcatheter aortic or mitral valve replacement, left ventricular assist device, venous arterial extracorporeal membrane oxygenation and transcatheter shunt closure.

It is imperative to investigate patients with cardiac prosthesis who develop anaemia. In addition to mechanical haemolytic anaemia, iron deficiency anaemia may occur due to chronic intravascular haemolysis or occult blood loss from the gastrointestinal tract because of coagulopathy secondary to warfarin intake. Elderly patients with co-morbidities may develop anaemia of chronic illness in which case anaemia is usually modest. The management of mechanic haemolytic anaemia entails correction of the underlying cardiac defects and iron and folate supplementation.

40.6   KEY POINTS

1. Defective valvular function should be considered in patients with mechanical valve replacement who develop hitherto unexplained anaemia.

2. Transoesophageal rather than transthoracic echocardiogram is often needed to delineate the valvular defects.

ADDITIONAL READING

1. Alkhouli, M, Farooq A, Go RS et al. Cardiac prosthesis related hemolytic anemia. Clin Cardiol 2019; 42: 692–700.

41 Paroxysmal Nocturnal Haemoglobinuria

41.1 CLINICAL SCENARIO

A 37-year-old man, who is a chronic smoker and social drinker, presented with a 1-month history of easy bruising, dizziness and breathlessness during mild exertion. Physical examination was unremarkable.

41.2 LABORATORY REPORTS

	Results	References	Units
Haemoglobin	9.5	13–17	g/dL
Mean corpuscular volume	104	82–95	fL
White cell count	2.33	4–10	10^9/L
Platelet count	28	150–400	10^9/L
Neutrophil count	0.74	2–7	10^9/L
Reticulocyte count	2.25	0.06–1.88	%
Lactate dehydrogenase	660	150–220	IU/L

Blood smear: No abnormal cells or dysplasia. Mild polychromasia. The patient's haemoglobin (Hb) concentration 6 months ago was 14.6 g/dL.

Liver and renal functions, serum vitamin B12 and folate were all within normal limits. Bone marrow showed mild trilineage hypoplasia with no dysplasia or abnormal cellular infiltration. Cytogenetics were normal. Immune markers including anti-nuclear antibody and rheumatoid factor were negative. Direct antiglobulin test was negative.

41.3 QUESTIONS

1. What is the next investigation?
2. What is the diagnosis?
3. What is the management plan?

41.4 CLINICAL PROGRESS

The presence of pancytopenia without abnormal marrow infiltration and the biochemical evidence of haemolysis with raised lactate dehydrogenase (LDH) led to the suspicion of paroxysmal nocturnal haemoglobinuria (PNH). Flow cytometric analysis was performed showing the presence of glycosylphosphatidylinositol (GPI)-deficient monocytes, neutrophils and red blood cells. A diagnosis of PNH was made. The patient was managed conservatively, but 2 months later, his Hb dropped to 6.2 g/dL, and platelet count has remained low at 20×10^9/L. He was managed as aplastic anaemia with cyclosporin A and eltrombopag with recovery of the platelet and white cell counts. However, repeated flow cytometric analyses showed progressive expansion of the PNH clone (Figure 41.1). Three years later, the patient presented with left calf pain, and doppler ultrasound confirmed left

DOI: 10.1201/9781003325413-48

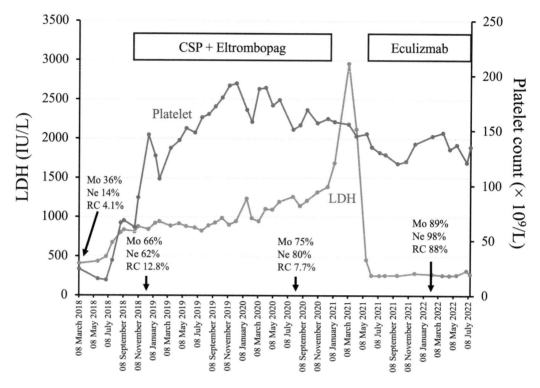

FIGURE 41.1 Haematological response and PNH clone size of a patient undergoing treatment with cyclosporin and eltrombopag and subsequently, eculizumab. CSP: Cyclosporin; LDH: Lactate dehydrogenase; Mo: Monocyte; Ne: Neutrophil: RC: Red Cell.

soleal vein thrombosis for which he received anticoagulation, and eltrombopag was stopped. At the same time, he complained of on-and-off dark urine, and his serum LDH rose to 2800 IU/L. He also complained of erectile dysfunction. He was treated with eculizumab with a prompt decrease in LDH. The PNH clone has now become the dominant haematopoietic clone.

41.5 PATHOGENESIS

PNH is an acquired clonal disorder of haematopoietic stem cells (HSC) arising from the somatic mutation of a gene encoding for phosphatidylinositol glycan anchor biosynthesis, class A (PIG-A). PIG-A is a glycosyl transferase responsible for the biosynthesis of a GPI anchor that attaches a subset of > 20 proteins to the surface of haematopoietic cells. In PNH, *PIG-A* mutations give rise to its loss of function, resulting in a variable reduction of GPI-anchored proteins, notably the complement inhibitory proteins CD55 (decay-accelerating factor [DAF]) and CD59 (membrane inhibitor of reactive lysis [MIRL]), which normally protect erythrocytes from the constitutively active alternative complement pathway. The alternative complement pathway includes two functional components, namely, complement C3 and C5 convertases that increase the formation of membrane attack complex (MAC), which is the final cytolytic event. Specifically, CD55 blocks the formation of the C3 and C5 convertases, whereas CD59 blocks the formation of MAC, primarily by inhibiting the binding and multiplicity of C9. Therefore, PNH cells lacking CD55 and CD59 become susceptible to complement-mediated cell lysis. The variable effects of *PIG-A* gene mutation on its function may account for the difference in penetrance. Red cells that are moderately sensitive (2–4 times) to complement activation are known as Type II, whereas those that are severely sensitive (15–25 times) are known as Type III cells. Red cells with normal sensitivity to complement activation are known as Type I cells.

41.6 CLINICAL MANIFESTATIONS

The clinical manifestations of PNH entail a triad of chronic intravascular haemolysis, bone marrow failure and thrombophilia. Although the pathogenetic mechanisms linking *PIG-A* mutations, complement activation and haemolysis have been well characterised, those about bone marrow failure and thrombophilia have remained unclear and speculative. PNH may also be identified in patients with marrow failure, particularly for those with aplastic anaemia, as part of the workup for pancytopenia. In this circumstance, haemolysis is mild or absent, and PNH clone size is mostly small (< 50%). In classical PNH, patients present with chronic intravascular haemolysis and haemoglobinuria, with biochemical evidence of haemolysis (raised LDH, unconjugated bilirubin and suppressed haptoglobin) and a large PNH clone as shown by > 50% GPI-deficient monocytes and neutrophils. High levels of haemoglobinaemia may result in smooth muscle dystonia, presenting with abdominal/back pain, oesophageal spasm and erectile dysfunction in males. Thrombosis is more common in patients with large PNH clones but may also occur in those with small clones. PNH-associated thrombosis is predominantly venous, but arterial thrombosis has also been reported. Abdominal veins are most commonly affected, but other sites can also be involved. Pathogenetic mechanisms of thrombosis are unclear, and both intravascular haemolysis and activation of PNH platelets may be involved. In our patient, PNH evolution was evident, suggesting that PNH can be viewed as a continuum ranging from marrow failure to overt intravascular haemolysis.

41.7 DIAGNOSIS

In most cases, PNH is diagnosed as part of the workup for pancytopenia in patients suspected of aplastic anaemia or clinically in patients with intravascular haemolysis. In aplastic anaemia, PNH screen may reveal small clones (< 50% GPI-deficient monocytes or neutrophils) in up to 50% of patients. Biochemical markers of haemolysis including LDH and bilirubin can be normal. In patients with clinical evidence of intravascular haemolysis and haemoglobinuria, serum LDH and bilirubin are raised, and haptoglobin is reduced. Direct antiglobulin test is negative. Reticulocyte count is raised but may be disproportionally low with respect to the degree of anaemia, indicating insufficient marrow activities. Bone marrow aspiration and biopsy are needed to ascertain marrow cellularity and morphologic features of myelodysplasia and detect abnormal cytogenetics and recurrent gene mutations associated with myelodysplastic syndrome. Flow cytometry typically shows large PNH clones (> 50%) in monocytes and neutrophils based on negative CD55 and CD59 expression. Erythrocytes are not reliable and may give rise to underestimation due to haemolysis of PNH clones and recent transfusion.

41.8 TREATMENT

Patients with aplastic anaemia and small PNH clones without intravascular haemolysis should be managed as aplastic anaemia, and no directed PNH therapy is needed. In contrast, patients with intravascular haemolysis suffer from constitutional and anaemic symptoms, haemoglobinaemia and risk of thrombosis and should receive PNH directed treatment. Eculizumab is a humanised monoclonal antibody that binds complement C5 and prevents its activation to C5b by C5 convertase of the alternative complement pathway, thereby inhibiting MAC formation. Eculizumab perturbs complement-mediated haemolysis in PNH, relieves associated symptoms and reduces risk of thrombosis. However, inhibition of the alternative complement pathway may increase the risk of infection, and vaccination against meningococcus is needed prior to treatment. Moreover, eculizumab has no apparent effect on PNH clone size, and long-term treatment is needed. Prophylaxis against venous thromboembolism is generally recommended. Other complement inhibitors targeting C5 and C3 are available. In case of an acute thrombotic event, anticoagulation with heparin or low-molecular-weight heparin is the first line of treatment. Direct oral anticoagulants are likely as effective as warfarin but have not been well studied in PNH.

41.9   KEY POINTS

1. PNH is an acquired clonal disorder of HSC arising from somatic mutation of the *PIG-A* gene.
2. PNH may present as bone marrow failure, intravascular haemolysis or thrombophilia, and patients should be managed accordingly.
3. Complement inhibitors are currently available for patients with severe haemolysis.

ADDITIONAL READINGS

1. Parker CJ. Update on the diagnosis and management of paroxysmal nocturnal hemoglobinuria. Hematology Am Soc Hematol Educ Program 2016; 2016(1): 208–216.
2. Brodsky RA. How I treat paroxysmal nocturnal hemoglobinuria. Blood 2021; 137(10): 1304–1309.

42 Thrombotic Thrombocytopenic Purpura

42.1 CLINICAL SCENARIO

A 47-year-old woman presented with symptomatic anaemia and expressive dysphasia for 1 day. Upon arrival to hospital, her temperature was 39°C, and she was mentally obtunded. There was no neck stiffness, lymphadenopathy or organomegaly. Her limb power and reflexes were normal.

42.2 LABORATORY REPORTS

	Results	References	Units
Haemoglobin	5.3	11.5–14.8	g/dL
White cell count	6.12	4–10	10^9/L
Platelet count	32	150–370	10^9/L
Creatinine	109	49–82	μmol/L
Bilirubin	41	4–23	μmol/L
Lactate dehydrogenase	1314	107–218	IU/L

Blood film showed leukoerythroblastic blood picture with prominent red cell fragments (9%, 2+) and mild polychromasia (Figure 42.1A, left panel). Her prothrombin time (PT)/activated partial thromboplastin time (APTT) was normal, and direct anti-globulin test (DAT) was negative. Brain computed tomography showed no evidence of intracranial bleeding or mass lesion.

42.3 QUESTIONS

1. What are the two main haematologic features?
2. What is the likely diagnosis?
3. What is the next investigation and management plan?

42.4 CLINICAL PROGRESS

The haematologic picture of hitherto unexplained microangiopathic haemolytic anaemia and thrombocytopenia has prompted investigations and management of thrombotic thrombocytopenic purpura (TTP). Both ADAMTS13 antibodies and activities were checked, and shortly thereafter, she underwent daily plasmapheresis. Methylprednisolone was also given at the same time. Her platelet count and lactate dehydrogenase (LDH) improved quickly after treatment and became normalised in 2 weeks (Figure 42.1A, right panel).

Laboratory results were available 3 days later, showing ADAMT13 activities of less than 5%, ADAMT13 antibody positive (> 90%) and ADAMT12 antigen less than 0.001 IU/mL. A diagnosis of TTP was made. Upon completion of plasma exchange, the patient received 4 weekly doses of rituximab (anti-CD20 monoclonal antibody). The ADAMTS13 activity became 71%, antibody level became 4.7% and antigen level was 0.849 IU/mL.

DOI: 10.1201/9781003325413-49

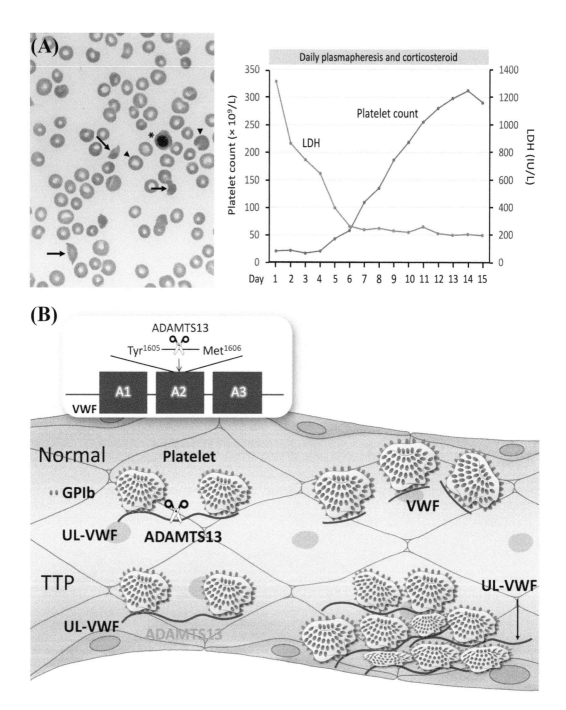

FIGURE 42.1 (A) (Left) Schistocytes (arrows), mild polychromasia (arrowheads), a nucleated red cell (asterisk) and thrombocytopenia in a thrombotic thrombocytopenic purpura (TTP) patient (Wright-Giemsa × 1000). (Right) Haematological responses to plasmapheresis and corticosteroid in a TTP patient. (B) Pathogenesis of TTP. ADAMTS13 cleaves the tyrosine methionine bond at the A2 domain of the ultra-large Von Willebrand Factor (UL-VWF) molecule and prevents platelet aggregation. Suppressed ADAMTS13 activity or the lack of it results in uncleaved UL-VWF, hence excessive platelet aggregation and microthrombi formation characteristic in TTP.

42.5 DIFFERENTIAL DIAGNOSIS OF THROMBOTIC MICROANGIOPATHY

Thrombotic microangiopathy (TMA) syndromes encompass a broad spectrum of diseases charac-terised by microangiopathic haemolytic anaemia (MAHA), thrombocytopenia and organ injury due to arteriolar and capillary thrombosis and the ensuing tissue ischaemia. In addition to TTP, which arises from defective or absent ADAMTS13 activities, other TMA syndromes are recognised. Complement-mediated TMA, also known as atypical haemolytic uraemic syndrome (aHUS) results from defective regulation of the alternative complement pathway due to underlying gene mutations affecting the regulatory or effector genes involved in the pathway. Autoantibodies targeting the complement pathway have also been reported. Acute kidney injury and hypertension are prominent features. Shiga toxin-mediated TMA, also known as ST-HUS, occurs mostly in children due to enteric infection by Shiga toxin-producing E. Coli, notably the O157:H7 strain or *S. dysenteriae*. The predominant symptoms are severe abdominal pain and bloody diarrhoea after intake of con-taminated food or water. Thrombocytopenia and acute kidney injury then ensue. Drug-related TMA can be due to drug-dependent antibody arising from quinine exposure or calcineurin inhibitors such as cyclosporin or tacrolimus because of endothelial dysfunction and increased platelet aggregation. Transplant-associated TMA is a distinct entity that occurs early in the course of haematopoietic stem cell transplantation and is characterised by endothelial injury and complement activation with normal ADAMTS13 activity. Trauma-associated TMA occurs in patients with severe and multiple blunt trauma, causing a release of Von Willebrand Factor (VWF) multimers from tissue endothe-lial cells. The prominent schistocytes distinguish it from disseminated intravascular coagulopathy (DIC) that may also occur in these clinical settings. In pregnant women, haemolysis (due to micro-angiopathy), elevated liver enzyme and low platelets, with the acronym **HELLP syndrome**, in the presence of hypertension and proteinuria, supported the diagnosis of pre-eclampsia.

42.6 PATHOGENESIS

In physiologic conditions, VWF multimers (including ultra-large VWF [UL-VWF]) that are syn-thesised in endothelial cells and platelets are released into the circulation upon activation of the endothelium. Under high shear stress, VWF multimers are extended and stretched in the direction of blood flow, unfolding the VWF A2 domain and exposing a cryptic Tyr-Met bond to be cleaved by ADAMTS13, which is synthesised by the liver. Such stress-induced proteolytic cleavage of VWF pre-vents microvascular thrombosis. In TTP, ADAMTS13 is absent or dysfunctional. Uncleaved UL-VWF multimers bind strongly to platelets, causing thrombosis and damage to red cells as the red cells pass through the perturbed microcirculation, hence the presence of schistocytes (Figure 42.1B). As the total volume of platelets in circulation of a normal adult is only 10–20 ml, sequestration of platelets due to formation of VWF–platelet aggregates uniformly gives rise to profound thrombocytopenia.

42.7 CLINICAL FEATURES

TTP is a rare disease, occurring in 1–5 cases per 1 million people per year. TTP is characterised pathologically by MAHA with severe thrombocytopenia. Patients may present with a myriad of clinical presentations, including fever, neurological symptoms, red–coloured urine due to haemo-globinuria or bleeding tendencies including petechiae and bruises. Renal impairment, if it happens, is usually mild. Chest discomfort can indicate myocardial ischaemia and may herald rapid clinical deterioration.

42.8 CAUSES

In 5% of cases, TTP is inherited and is known as Upshaw–Schulman syndrome due to bi-allelic mutations of the *ADAMTS13* gene. In 95% of cases, ADAMTS13 deficiency is due to autoantibod-ies targeting ADAMTS13. Acquired TTP can be categorised into primary, when no underlying cause can be identified, or secondary when it is associated with underlying diseases, including human immunodeficiency virus infection and autoimmune disease, particularly systemic lupus erythematosus.

42.9 INVESTIGATIONS

The presence of MAHA and thrombocytopenia should prompt the investigation for TTP. Typically, DAT is negative, and the PT, APTT and fibrinogen level are normal. The D-dimer level is raised. ADAMTS13 activity, now the gold standard for the diagnosis of TTP, is essential. The assay is based on degradation of full–length VWF or synthetic peptides of VWF by ADAMTS13 in patients' plasma, and the cleavage products are detected primarily by fluorescence resonance energy transfer (FRET). Anti-ADAMTS13 autoantibodies, predominantly immunoglobulin G that is present in most acquired but not inherited TTP, can be readily detected by enzyme-linked immunosorbent assay (ELISA). Two types of autoantibodies are known: inhibitory antibodies neutralise the proteolytic activity of ADAMTS13, and non-inhibitory antibodies bind ADAMTS13 and increase its plasma clearance. In both cases, autoantibodies are polyclonal and show broad specificity against all domains of ADAMTS13. ADAMTS13 antigen can be measured by ELISA, but this is not routinely measured.

42.10 MANAGEMENT APPROACH

TTP is considered a medical emergency. Patients with hitherto unexplained MAHA and thrombocytopenia should receive **plasmapheresis** immediately before an ADAMTS13 activity result is available. In this process, autoantibodies are removed, and normal ADAMTS13 is replenished from fresh frozen plasma or cryoreduced plasma (CRP). Plasmapheresis is performed daily until normalisation of the platelet count and LDH. Simultaneously, **corticosteroid** is given to suppress production of autoantibodies by B- and plasma cells. Typically, a corticosteroid dose is tapered over 3–4 weeks. Along the same line, anti-CD20 monoclonal antibody **rituximab** has been used at the completion of plasmapheresis to suppress autoantibodies production by B-cells and hence reduce disease relapse. It is usually given in weekly doses for 4 weeks. In patients who are refractory or who relapse after treatment, **alternative immunosuppression and splenectomy** may be considered. New therapeutic agents are on the horizon. Specifically, **caplacizumab**, a humanised immunoglobulin targeting the A1 domain of VWF has been approved for the treatment of TTP in conjunction with plasmapheresis and immunosuppression. It blocks the interaction between VWF and platelets, hence preventing microvascular thrombi formation.

42.11 KEY POINTS

1. Patients with hitherto unexplained MAHA and thrombocytopenia should be investigated for TTP, which is a medical emergency, and treated with plasmapheresis until laboratory results confirm otherwise.
2. TTP is caused by deficient ADAMTS13 activities, which in most cases, results from autoantibodies against ADAMTS13.
3. In addition to plasmapheresis, TTP treatment includes corticosteroid and rituximab, and for relapsed or refractory cases, alternative immunosuppressant and splenectomy should be considered.

ADDITIONAL READINGS

1. George JN, Nester CM. Syndromes of thrombotic microangiopathy. N Engl J Med 2014; 371: 654–666.
2. Sukumar S, Lämmle B, Cataland SR. Thrombotic thrombocytopenic purpura: pathophysiology, diagnosis, and management. J Clin Med 2021; 10: 536.

43 Atypical Haemolytic Uraemic Syndrome

43.1 CLINICAL SCENARIO

A 32-year-old woman, a carrier of α thalassaemia, was admitted to hospital for delivery of a pair of identical twins. Except for the known hypochromic microcytic anaemia (Haemoglobin 10 g/dL, White cell count 8.0×10^9/L, Platelet count 170×10^9/L), her blood tests were unremarkable before delivery. One day after delivery, she complained of shortness of breath.

43.2 LABORATORY REPORTS

43.2.1 HAEMATOLOGY

	Results	References	Units
Haemoglobin	6.9	11.7–14.8	g/dL
Mean corpuscular volume	63.9	82–96	fL
Mean corpuscular haemoglobin	20.4	27.5–33.2	pg
White cell count	21.7	4.4–10.1	10^9/L
Platelet count	53	17–380	10^9/L
Reticulocyte count	4.02	0.5–2.5	%
D-dimer	7273	0.5–500	mg/L FEU*

* FEU: Fibrinogen Equivalent Unit.
Prothrombin time/Activated partial thromboplastin time: Normal. Liver enzymes: Normal.
Blood film: Presence of nucleated red cells, polychromasia and schistocytes (Figure 43.1).

43.2.2 BIOCHEMISTRY

	Results	References	Units
Sodium	133	136–148	mmol/L
Potassium	6.3	3.6–5.0	mmol/L
Creatinine	235	49–82	μmol/L
Lactate dehydrogenase	700	100–250	IU/L
Haptoglobin	0.088	0.32–1.97	g/L

43.3 QUESTIONS

1. What are the possible diagnoses?
2. What further investigations should be performed?
3. What is the management plan?

DOI: 10.1201/9781003325413-50

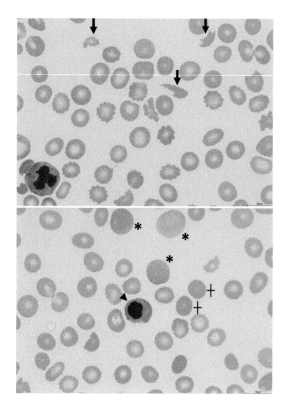

FIGURE 43.1 Characteristic microangiopathic haemolytic anaemia and thrombocytopenia in atypical hae-molytic uraemic syndrome. Arrows: Schistocytes; Asterisks: Polychromasia; Arrowhead: Nucleated red cells; Cross: Spherocytes. Platelets were not encountered in this field.

43.4   CLINICAL PROGRESS

The haematological picture was that of microangiopathic haemolytic anaemia and thrombocyto-penia. Direct antiglobulin test was negative, and autoimmune haemolytic anaemia was unlikely. Serum ADAMTS13 activity was 15%, falling short of the 10% cutoff characteristic of thrombotic thrombocytopenic purpura (TTP). ADAMTS13 antibody was negative. Therefore, TTP was also unlikely. A diagnosis of atypical haemolytic uraemic syndrome (aHUS) was made. Gene mutations associated with aHUS and anti-Factor H autoantibody were negative. She received eculizumab weekly for 4 weeks followed by every 2 weeks. Platelet count and serum lactate dehydrogenase returned to normal in 2 weeks.

43.5   THROMBOTIC MICROANGIOPATHY DURING PREGNANCY

Thrombotic microangiopathy during pregnancy is a serious complication as it may be associated with potentially life–threatening conditions. Differential diagnoses include TTP, aHUS, dissemi-nated intravascular coagulopathy (DIC), HELLP syndrome/acute fatty liver of pregnancy and eclampsia.

43.6   HAEMOLYTIC URAEMIC SYNDROME

Haemolytic uraemic syndrome (HUS) is a heterogenous group of diseases characterised clinically by **non-immune microangiopathic haemolytic anaemia**, **thrombocytopenia** and **acute kidney**

injury. The pathological process entails **endothelial damage**, microthrombi formation in multiple organs, platelet consumption and intravascular mechanical haemolysis. It is different from TTP, which is caused by acquired or congenital deficiency of ADAMTS13 (a disintegrin and metalloproteinase with thrombospondin–type 1 motifs, member 13), a Von Willebrand protease that breaks down Von Willebrand multimers. Pathological features in HUS reflect tissue responses to endothelial injury, including endothelial swelling, subendothelial widening and the presence of luminal fibrin with entrapped and fragmented red cells. In kidney tissue, substantial luminal occlusion in glomerular capillaries and arterioles can occur. Ultrastructural evaluation shows glomerular endothelial swelling, fenestral fusion, subendothelial expansion with electron–lucent material and later reduplication of the glomerular basement membrane.

43.7   CLASSIFICATION

Based on aetiology, HUS can be broadly classified into infection–associated and atypical HUS. **Infection–associated HUS** is caused by Shiga toxin–producing *Escherichia coli* (STEC), *Streptococcus pneumoniae* and H1N1/influenza A. **Atypical HUS** (aHUS) can be primary or secondary. Primary aHUS is associated with complement gene mutation or Factor H autoantibodies, leading to complement activation. Mutations of genes associated with cobalamin metabolism (methylmalonic aciduria and homocystinuria type C protein [*MMACHC*]), intracellular signaling (diacylglycerol kinase epsilon [*DGKE*]) and cellular differentiation (Wilm's tumour 1 [*WT1*]) have also been reported. Secondary aHUS can be caused by infection, malignant hypertension, complement amplifying conditions such as systemic lupus erythematosus, scleroderma and antiphospholipid syndrome, pregnancy, stem cell and solid organ transplantation and drugs such as calcineurin inhibitors, oral contraceptives and quinine. Patients with apparently secondary aHUS could also have a co-existing genetic predisposition frequently encountered in primary aHUS. In both primary and secondary aHUS, uncontrolled activation of the alternate complement pathway results in tissue damage.

43.8   DIAGNOSIS

A high index of suspicion and early diagnosis of HUS are critical to reduce morbidity and prevent mortality. The triad of non-immune microangiopathic haemolytic anaemia, thrombocytopenia and acute kidney injury is characteristic and should raise clinical suspicion. Clinical and family history, age at presentation, recent illnesses and associated symptoms guide subsequent evaluations. aHUS is primarily a diagnosis of exclusion, and differential diagnoses including consumptive coagulopathy and TTP should be considered.

43.9   MANAGEMENT

Specific management depends on the causative factors. In pregnancy–associated aHUS, uncontrolled complement activation occurs during pregnancy or post-partum. In contrast to eclampsia or HELLP syndrome, which typically subside after delivery, pregnancy–associated aHUS may persist and progress post-partum. In the pre-eculizumab era, most patients progressed to end–stage renal failure. Currently, therapy targeting complement activation has become the mainstay of treatment. Eculizumab is a humanised monoclonal immunoglobulin G antibody that binds to the C5 complement protein and blocks its cleavage, thereby preventing the formation of C5b-9, the membrane attack complex. Other monoclonal antibodies that block complement activation have also been approved. The optimal duration of eculizumab treatment is presently unknown. The extremely high cost and risk of infection due to suppression of the complement pathway might hamper long–term treatment with eculizumab. However, there are concerns about relapse after discontinuation of treatment. Plasmapheresis used to be the mainstay of treatment before the eculizumab era but is now replaced by eculizumab, except when eculizumab is not available.

43.10   KEY POINTS

1. HUS is clinically characterised by non-immune microangiopathic haemolytic anaemia, thrombocytopenia and acute kidney injury.
2. Complement activation is the main pathogenesis in most cases of HUS.
3. HUS can be broadly classified into infection–associated and atypical HUS. Primary atypical HUS is characterised by gene mutations. Secondary atypical aHUS is associated with a wide range of clinical conditions, including pregnancy.
4. Therapy targeting complement activation, notably eculizumab, is the mainstay of treatment for aHUS.

ADDITIONAL READING

1. Michael M, Bagga A, Sartain SE, Smith RJ. Haemolytic uraemic syndrome. Lancet 2022; 400: 1722–1740.

Thrombocytopenia

44 Immune Thrombocytopenia

44.1 CLINICAL SCENARIO

A 30-year-old woman with good past health presented with easy bruising for 1 month. She was married and had no children. Her mother had systemic lupus erythematosus on a low dose of immunosuppression. Physical examination showed petechiae in both legs and a few bruises.

44.2 LABORATORY REPORTS

	Results	References	Units
Haemoglobin	14.4	11.5–14.8	g/dL
White cell count	6.22	3.89–9.93	10^9/L
Platelet count	6	167–396	10^9/L
Prothrombin time	12.2	11.3–13.5	Seconds
Activated partial thromboplastin time	28.1	25.9–33.7	Seconds

Blood film: Genuine thrombocytopenia. Giant platelets were present. Normal differential count.
Liver and renal function tests: Unremarkable.

44.3 QUESTIONS

1. What is the likely diagnosis?
2. What additional investigations are needed?
3. What is the management plan?

44.4 CLINICAL PROGRESS

Further investigations showed anti-nuclear antibody titre of 1/80. Anti-double stranded DNA antibody and the panel of anti-extractable nuclear antigen antibody were negative. Direct Monoclonal Antibody-specific Immobilisation of Platelet Antigen (MAIPA) showed the presence of autoantibodies against platelet glycoprotein IIb/IIIa on the patient's platelets. Indirect MAIPA also showed free antibodies against platelet glycoprotein Ia/IIa and Ib/IX. Bone marrow (BM) aspiration showed normal haemopoiesis with a mild increase in megakaryocytes that showed normal morphology. A diagnosis of immune thrombocytopenia (ITP) was made. The patient was given prednisolone and intravenous immunoglobulin (IVIG), and her platelet count became normalised in 2 weeks. However, as her steroid was being tapered, her platelet count dropped suddenly on week 4 of steroid treatment; she was given eltrombopag, and her platelet count became normal again, which was stable upon cessation of the steroid.

44.5 CLINICAL FEATURES

ITP is defined by the presence of hitherto unexplained thrombocytopenia with a platelet count of less than 100×10^9/L. It is a diagnosis by exclusion. In adults, ITP often shows an insidious and apparently unprovoked onset. ITP may be a primary condition or it may have other causes, including drugs (e.g., rifampicin and vancomycin), lymphoproliferative disease (e.g., chronic lymphocytic

DOI: 10.1201/9781003325413-52

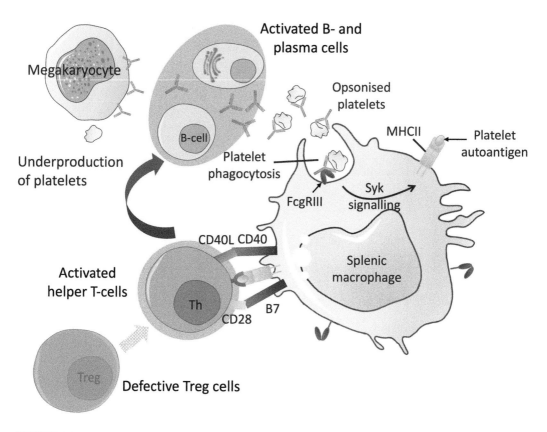

FIGURE 44.1   Pathogenesis of immune thrombocytopenia (ITP). Both opsonisation of platelets and suppression of platelet release from megakaryocytes by autoantibody contribute to thrombocytopenia. Generation of autoantibody from activated B- and plasma cells arises from helper T-cell activation, secondary to antigen presentation from splenic macrophage and defective regulatory T-cells. MHCII: Major histocompatibility complex class II; FcgRIII: Fc gamma receptor III; Syk: Spleen tyrosine kinase; Th: Helper T-cell; Treg: Regulatory T-cell.

leukaemia), an immunodeficient state (e.g., common variable immunodeficiency [CVID]), infection (e.g., human immunodeficiency virus [HIV] and *Helicobacter pylori*) and autoimmune disease (e.g., systemic lupus erythematosus and anti-phospholipid syndrome). The incidence of ITP shows a bi-modal pattern: one peak of incidence between 20 and 30 years of age with a slight female predominance and a larger peak after 60 years of age with equal sex distribution. Despite effective treatment (see the following) and initial response, relapse is common, and chronic ITP develops in up to 70% of adults with this condition.

44.6   PATHOGENESIS

ITP is an organ-specific autoimmune disease characterised by both increased platelet destruction and relative platelet underproduction that collectively result in thrombocytopenia. For a long time, the presence of **anti-platelet autoantibody** was thought to be core to ITP pathogenesis, with the antibody-coated platelets being recognised by the splenic macrophages via the Fc gamma receptors III (FcgRIII), leading to platelet phagocytosis and destruction (Figure 44.1).

It is increasingly recognised that anti-platelet autoantibody is released from autoreactive B-cells that arise from the loss of self-tolerance. This is due to **defective CD4+ regulatory T-cell (Treg) production** that normally modulates helper T-cells and dendritic cells to function; as a result, both populations become unopposed, leading to B-cell activation and increased antigen presentation, respectively. In fact, the macrophages as antigen-presenting cells also become activated, and they present platelet autoantigens to T helper cells via major histocompatibility complex class II molecules, generating an autoantigen feedback loop. The immunoglobulin G (IgG) autoantibodies bind to platelet surface glycoproteins. On the one hand, they are directly recognised by macrophages in the spleen, and on the other hand, IgG may fix complement, generating complement fragments that opsonise the platelets. In both circumstances, platelets become phagocytosed, resulting in thrombocytopenia. Binding of autoantibody to megakaryocytes in BM may induce apoptosis, leading to platelet underproduction. Emerging evidence shows that cytotoxic T-cell activation may also inhibit the production of platelets.

44.7   DIAGNOSIS

The diagnosis of ITP is by exclusion. Specifically, a thorough **drug history** should exclude iatrogenic causes of thrombocytopenia with notable examples being antibiotics, anti-tuberculosis medication and heparin. Amidst **critical illness and sepsis**, disseminated intravascular coagulopathy or thrombotic thrombocytopenic purpura should be ruled out. Patients with Dengue fever can also present with profound thrombocytopenia akin to ITP. In patients who show a long history of refractory "ITP", **hereditary causes** of thrombocytopenia should be considered. Patients with evidence of lymphadenopathy or hepatosplenomegaly should be investigated for underlying **haematological malignancies** that may present as isolated thrombocytopenia. Patients in the third trimester of **pregnancy** typically develop modest thrombocytopenia due to dilutional effects, also known as gestational thrombocytopenia.

Conditions associated with ITP should be identified. Signs and symptoms related to underlying autoimmune diseases particularly systemic lupus erythematosus should be evaluated in young female patients. Serological tests should be performed. A history of venereal exposure in male patients who present with isolated thrombocytopenia should raise the suspicion of ITP associated with HIV infection, and anti-HIV-1/-2 antibody should be tested.

Careful blood film examination is essential. The presence of platelet clumps, especially in asymptomatic patients, should prompt the diagnosis of erroneous thrombocytopenia. In patients with *bona fide* ITP, thrombocytopenia, with or without the presence of giant platelets, should be the only abnormality. Hereditary causes of thrombocytopenia may be revealed as abnormal platelet morphology, known as hereditary megathrombocytopenia. Unexplained abnormalities in white cell or erythroid series should prompt investigations for underlying marrow pathology. Except in elderly or unfit patients, BM examination should be performed to rule out BM pathologies. Abnormalities in renal and liver functions should also prompt the investigation of alternative diagnoses.

The diagnostic and prognostic values of demonstrating autoantibodies have remained controversial, and the assays have not been universally adopted. The MAIPA assay can detect autoantibodies that are bound directly on the platelet surface (direct MAIPA) or indirectly in the plasma (indirect MAIPA). A positive MAIPA assay can be used to support a diagnosis of ITP although a negative result does not rule out the diagnosis.

44.8   MANAGEMENT

The risk of life-threatening bleeding and hence the benefit of treatment should be weighed against the side effects of treatment. In general, patients without bleeding and platelet $\geq 30 \times 10^9$/L should be closely monitored. Those with signs of bleedings or platelet $< 20 \times 10^9$/L should receive treatment. Mechanistically, medical treatments aim at reducing autoantibody production, increasing platelet production, blocking antibody bound platelet to macrophage FcgRIII receptors, preventing macrophage internalisation and clearance of opsonised platelets (Figure 44.1).

Corticosteroid is the first-line treatment, and typically, platelet count responds in a few days. Once the platelet count has become normal, the dose should be tapered gradually over a period of 6 weeks to avoid toxicity of long-term steroids. Patients with refractory, relapsed or steroid-dependent diseases should receive second-line therapy. In the past, splenectomy was the standard of care, resulting in rapid recovery of platelet count in most patients, but relapses occur in nearly 50% of them. However, there is associated risk of complications, particularly post-operative abdominal vein thrombosis and infection by encapsulated bacteria. Presently, these patients are mostly treated by **thrombopoietin (TPO) mimetics** including eltrombopag or romiplostim or **monoclonal antibody against CD20**. Eltrombopag is a small molecule that binds to the transmembrane portion of the TPO receptor. Romiplostim is a large peptibody molecule that binds to the same site as native TPO on the extracellular domain of the TPO receptor. These novel agents have largely replaced immunosuppressive agents, including azathioprine, mycophenolate mofetil or cyclosporin, as well as androgen danazol, which was once used frequently for this disease.

In situations where a rapid rise in platelet count is needed due to bleeding and profound thrombocytopenia, **IVIG** can be used. This is a human-derived blood product comprising mainly IgG, and it works by binding to the Fc receptor of macrophage, sparing the binding of antibody-coated platelets. Platelet transfusion, unless in a life-threatening bleeding situation, is usually not warranted due to its extremely short half-life in ITP patients.

A number of new treatments are currently available in ITP patients who fail first- and second-line treatment. Fostamatinib inhibits spleen tyrosine kinase (SYK) that is involved in the destruction of antibody-coated platelets in macrophage. Avatrombopag is a small molecule that binds to the same site as eltrombopag and stimulates the production of platelets by megakaryocytes. Other agents that are now in clinical trials for ITP treatment include the inhibitor of neonatal Fc receptor, which is normally expressed in the endothelial cells and assists in the recycling of phagocytosed IgG. The recycling process is blocked by the inhibitor, leading to impaired recycling and a reduced serum level of autoantibodies. Bruton's tyrosine kinase inhibitor inhibits B-cell activities and is currently indicated for the treatment of B-cell malignancies; reduced B-cell activities may in principle reduce the production of autoantibody. Monoclonal antibody reduces the binding of B-cell activating factor (BAFF) to B-cells and may also reduce the production of autoantibodies. Agents currently indicated for the treatment of multiple myeloma, including anti-CD38 antibody and proteasome inhibitor bortezomib, are being evaluated for the treatment of ITP.

44.9   KEY POINTS

1. ITP is a diagnosis by exclusion and is characterised by increased platelet destruction and relative platelet underproduction.
2. ITP results from anti-platelet autoantibodies released by autoreactive B-cells due to the loss of self-tolerance because of defective CD4+ regulatory T-cells.
3. Treatment is indicated for patients with bleeding or profound thrombocytopenia. Corticosteroid is the first-line treatment. Rituximab and TPO mimetics are the second line. IVIG may induce a transient rise in platelet count. Platelet transfusion is ineffective, except for life-threatening bleeding conditions.

ADDITIONAL READINGS

1. Provan D, Semple JW. Recent advances in the mechanisms and treatment of immune thrombocytopenia. eBioMedicine 2022; 76: 103820.
2. Semple JW, Rebetz J, Maouia A, Kapur R. An update on the pathophysiology of immune thrombocytopenia. Curr Opin Hematol 2020; 27: 423–429.
3. Kuter DJ. Novel therapies for immune thrombocytopenia. Br J Haematol 2022; 196: 1311–1328.

45 Hereditary Macrothrombocytopenia

45.1 CLINICAL SCENARIO

A 22-year-old woman with a history of cataract had check-up prior to tonsillectomy. She has regular menstruation with normal cycle and flow. Her mother also had cataract and bone marrow examination a long time ago for thrombocytopenia and was diagnosed "immune thrombocytopenia", but treatment has never been effective. Her elder brother suffered from deafness and renal failure on continuous ambulatory peritoneal dialysis (CAPD).

45.2 LABORATORY REPORTS

	Results	References	Units
Haemoglobin	14.3	11.5–14.8	g/dL
White cell count	4.7	3.89–9.93	10^9/L
Platelet count	24	167–396	10^9/L

Blood smear: No platelet clump. Presence of giant platelets. Normal red cell morphology. White cells showed normal differential. A few neutrophils showed bluish inclusion (Figure 45.1).

45.3 QUESTIONS

1. What are the further investigations?
2. What is the likely diagnosis?
3. What is the management plan?

45.4 CLINICAL PROGRESS

Flow cytometry of the platelet showed normal immunophenotype. Platelet function assay (PFA-100) upon exposure to epinephrine and adenosine diphosphate (ADP) was normal. The patient was given platelet transfusion before and during the operation with no excessive bleeding. Subsequent genetic mutation tests confirmed the presence of a pathogenic *MYH9* V1516L mutation in exon 31. A diagnosis of hereditary macrothrombocytopenia due to *MYH9*-related disease was made.

45.5 HEREDITARY MACROTHROMBOCYTOPENIA—CLINICAL SPECTRUM

Hereditary macrothrombocytopenia belongs to the family of hereditary thrombocytopenia, which is a growing list of diseases as more gene mutations are identified by next generation sequencing. To date, more than 30 gene mutations that are involved in megakaryopoiesis and platelet generation have been reported. In particular, *MYH9* is the most frequently mutated gene in these diseases. It encodes the heavy chain of non-muscle myosin IIA, which interacts with actin filaments to generate the mechanical forces needed for proplatelet formation, fragmentation and platelet release. The diseases are known collectively as *MYH9*–related disease (*MYH9*–RD).

DOI: 10.1201/9781003325413-53

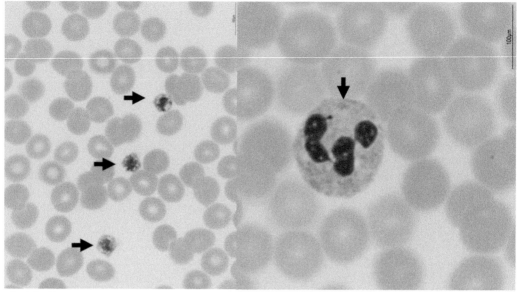

CTCCAAGGATGATGTGGGCAAGAGTGT
                    T

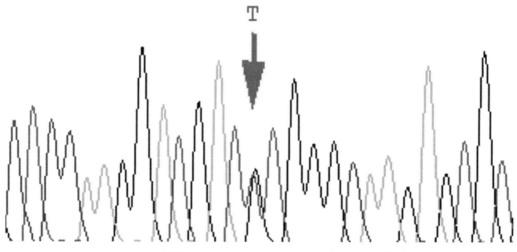

Exon 31 mutation at codon 1516
(*G*TG→*T*TG; val→leu) or V1516L

FIGURE 45.1 (Left upper) Blood film showing giant platelets (arrows). (Right upper) Neutrophils showing bluish cytoplasmic inclusion (arrow). (Lower) DNA sequencing showing the pathogenic *MYH9* V1516L mutation in exon 31.

MYH9–RD is caused by monoallelic mutations in *MYH9* and is inherited as an autosomal dominant disorder. Patients typically present at birth with giant platelets, thrombocytopenia and neutrophil inclusion. Bleeding tendency, if any, is mostly mild. In some patients, macrothrombocytopenia is the only manifestation. Sensorineural hearing loss is common, ranging from a mild defect to profound deafness. In about one-third of patients, nephropathy ensues, leading to end-stage renal disease. About 20% of patients suffer from presenile cataracts.

45.6 DIAGNOSIS

Patients with hereditary macrothrombocytopenia usually present with a long history of thrombocytopenia and associated diseases. Further investigations are initiated by the presence of characteristic giant platelets and neutrophil inclusion bodies in blood smear and a family history of thrombocytopenia and syndromal diseases. In the past, *in vitro* platelet aggregation and flow cytometry for platelet immunophenotype would be performed to rule out alternative diagnoses, and immunofluorescence for MYH9 protein aggregates in neutrophils would suggest *MYH9*–RD. At present, definitive diagnosis of hereditary macrothrombocytopenia can be confirmed by genetic testing.

45.7 CLINICAL RELEVANCE

An important differential diagnosis is immune thrombocytopenia. The distinction is clinically important as the treatment used for the latter is ineffective and potentially toxic for hereditary macrothrombocytopenia. In addition, patients with hereditary macrothrombocytopenia secondary to *ANKRD26*, *ETV6* and *RUNX1* are at risk of myeloid malignancy due to germline predisposition. Precise genetic information is essential for genetic counselling. Furthermore, patients with *MYH9*–RD are associated with syndromal manifestations, and early intervention may ameliorate the clinical severity of these diseases.

Patients with hereditary macrothrombocytopenia who present with bleeding should be managed by supportive platelet transfusion and antifibrinolytic agents and in severe cases, activated Factor VII. Off-label use of thrombopoietin mimetics has been reported in anecdotal cases.

45.8 KEY POINTS

1. Consider inherited thrombocytopenia in patients with unexplained thrombocytopenia.
2. Patients with *MYH9*–RD show macrothrombocytopenia and bluish cytoplasmic inclusion of neutrophils associated with cataract, hearing defects and nephropathy.

ADDITIONAL READINGS

1. Noris P, Pecci A. Hereditary thrombocytopenias: a growing list of disorders. Hematology Am Soc Hematol Educ Program 2017; 2017(1): 385–399.
2. Collins J, Astle WJ, Megy K, Mumford AD, Vuckovic D. Advances in understanding the pathogenesis of hereditary macrothrombocytopenia. Br J Haematol 2021; 195: 25–45.

Miscellaneous Conditions

46 Castleman Disease

46.1 CLINICAL SCENARIO

A 37-year-old administrator presented with malaise, night sweats and weight loss of 8 kg (baseline body weight 90 kg) for 1 month in March 2022. He was married with no children. He was a single child, and there was no family history of blood diseases or malignancies. Except for hyperlipidaemia and gout, he has enjoyed remarkable past health. Physical examination showed enlarged lymph nodes at about 2 cm at the left axilla and right groin. There was no organomegaly. Positron emission tomography/Computed tomography (PET/CT) showed generalised, mildly hypermetabolic and enlarged lymph nodes. There was increased uptake in bone marrow.

46.2 LABORATORY REPORTS

	Results	References	Units
Haemoglobin	11.2	11.5–14.8	g/dL
White cell count	9.9	3.89–9.93	10^9/L
Platelet count	454	167–396	10^9/L
Erythrocyte sedimentation rate	116	< 15	mm/hr
C-reactive protein	10.3	< 0.5	mg/dL
Globulin	60	24–36	g/L

46.3 QUESTIONS

1. What is the next investigation?
2. What are the possible diagnoses?
3. What are the principles of management?

46.4 CLINICAL PROGRESS

Excisional biopsy of the right groin lymph node was performed, showing reactive lymphoid hyperplasia with germinal centre regression and prominent polytypic plasmacytic proliferation with areas of a sheet-like pattern (Figures 46.1A–46.1C). The immunoglobulin (Ig) G4+ to IgG+ plasma cells' ratio was 20%. Human Herpesvirus-8 (HHV-8) and Epstein-Barr virus-encoded RNA (EBER) immunostaining were negative. Bone marrow showed reactive plasmacytosis with no abnormal infiltration. His serum IgG and IgM measured 3875 (Ref: 650–1620 mg/dL) and 438 (Ref: 50–300 mg/dL), respectively. Serum IgG4 was 2.4 g/L (Ref: 0.04–0.86 g/L). Serum anti-human immunodeficiency virus (HIV) antibody was negative. A diagnosis of multicentric Castleman disease was made. He received tocilizumab once every 2 weeks and his C-reactive protein returned to normal level (Figure 46.1D).

46.5 CASTLEMAN DISEASE

Castleman disease (CD) comprises a heterogeneous group of diseases characterised by inflammatory lymphadenopathy with specific histological features. Clinically, it can be classified as unicentric (UCD) or multicentric (MCD) CD. **UCD** involves a single lymph node or group of lymph nodes with histological feature of a hyaline-vascular subtype (80–90%), and the disease typically

DOI: 10.1201/9781003325413-55

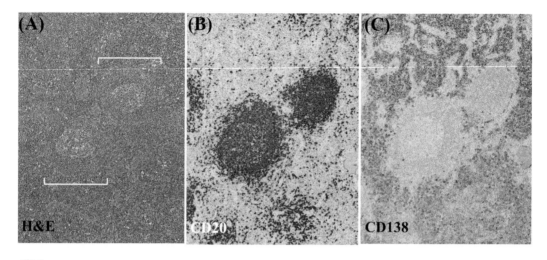

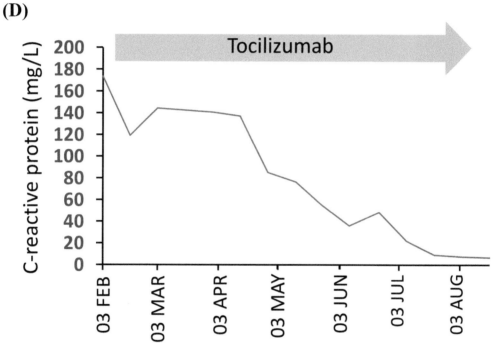

FIGURE 46.1 (A) H&E: The lymph node showing preserved nodal architecture. The interfollicular areas were expanded and characterised by mature plasma cells and prominent vasculature. (B) The lymphoid follicles were shown by CD20+ mature B-cells. (C) The interfollicular areas were highlighted by CD138+ plasma cells. (D) Treatment response to interleukin-6 receptor antagonist tocilizumab based on the serum level of C-reactive protein. (*Figures 46.1A–46.1C, courtesy of Dr. Wong Shun.*)

runs an indolent course without systemic symptoms. About 10–20% UCD lymphadenopathy shows features of the plasmacytic subtype, and these patients often present with systemic symptoms (see the following). UCD is associated with paraneoplastic pemphigus (PNP), bronchiolitis obliterans (BO), Amyloid A amyloidosis, vascular neoplasms and possibly lymphomas. **MCD** can be classified as human HHV-8–associated MCD, POEMS–associated MCD, and idiopathic MCD (iMCD). Histologically, most MCD shows features of the plasmacytic subtype. In most cases of MCD, patients present with systemic inflammatory symptoms, including fever, weight loss, generalised oedema, lymphadenopathy and hepatosplenomegaly. Organ dysfunction may occur, which may progress rapidly. HHV-8–associated MCD is most commonly seen in HIV-infected patients. In POEMS–associated MCD, peripheral neuropathy, organomegaly, endocrinopathy, monoclonal paraproteins and skin changes may be present. A subset of iMCD, known as TAFRO, manifests with thrombocytopenia, ascites, fever, reticulin fibrosis and organomegaly.

46.6   DIAGNOSIS

Diagnosis of CD is based on histological features of lymphadenopathy. Excision biopsy is advisable for diagnosis and exclusion of differential diagnoses. PET/CT scan is needed to ascertain the extent of lymphadenopathy. Virological and rheumatological investigations for HHV-8, HIV and autoimmune causes of lymphadenopathy are essential. The serum IgG4 level should be examined. Differential diagnoses include lymphoma, IgG4-related diseases, viral infections by Epstein–Barr virus, cytomegalovirus or HIV and autoimmune and reactive causes of lymphadenopathy. The increase in the IgG4 level and IgG4+ to IgG+ plasma cells fell short of the criteria for IgG4-related disease in the present case, and together with the predominance of prototypic plasma cells, the histological features of the patient's case were more consistent with those of iMCD.

46.7   MANAGEMENT

UCD that is resectable should be surgically excised, and > 90% of patients survive beyond 5 years. Relapse is relatively rare, and associated symptoms usually resolve after surgery. Unresectable UCD can be treated with rituximab with or without steroids followed by surgical resection or radiotherapy. iMCD is treated by monoclonal antibody therapies directed at interleukin (IL)-6 (siltuximab) and its receptor (tocilizumab). The clinical responses in iMCD attest to the important role of IL-6 signaling in its pathogenesis. The most common adverse effects with siltuximab are pruritus and upper respiratory tract infections, whilst with tocilizumab, the most common adverse effects are elevated transaminases (30%) and hyperlipidaemia (20%). Rituximab is advocated as second-line treatment for refractory cases, and in severe cases, a combination cytotoxic chemotherapy using either lymphoma or myeloma regimens can be effective. Efficacy of mTOR and JAK inhibitors has been reported. With these treatments, the 5-year overall survival was estimated to be > 70% and > 95% among the responders. HHV-8-associated MCD, particularly for patients with concurrent Kaposi sarcoma, may respond to a rituximab-based chemotherapy regimen. In fact, such patients may develop lymphoma, particularly primary effusion or plasmablastic lymphoma. Patients with HIV infection should also receive anti-retroviral therapy. POEMS–associated MCD should be treated for POEMS.

46.8   KEY POINTS

1. CD is characterised by inflammatory lymphadenopathy. Clinically, it includes unicentric (UCD) and multicentric variants (MCD).
2. MCD is associated with HHV-8 and POEMS. Other cases are idiopathic and known as iMCD.
3. The mainstay of treatment for iMCD is about targeting IL-6 receptors or ligands.

ADDITIONAL READINGS

1. Rhee FV, Oksenhendler E, Srkalovic G et al. International evidence-based consensus diagnostic and treatment guidelines for unicentric castleman disease. Blood Adv 2020; 4(23): 5039–6050.
2. Carbone A, Borok M, Damania B et al. Castleman disease. Nat Rev Dis Primers 2021; 7(84): 1–18.

47 Haemophagocytic Lymphohistiocytosis

47.1 CLINICAL SCENARIO

A 28-year-old woman with good past health presented with fever and myalgia for two days. She was a single child in the family and worked as a receptionist. There was no family history of blood diseases or malignancies. She was jaundiced, and there was no rash, lymphadenopathy or organomegaly.

47.2 LABORATORY REPORTS

47.2.1 HAEMATOLOGY

	Results	References	Units
Haemoglobin	13.9	11.5–14.8	g/dL
White cell count	1.8	3.89–9.93	10^9/L
Neutrophil count	1.55	2.01–7.42	10^9/L
Lymphocyte count	0.22	1.06–3.61	10^9/L
Platelet count	20	167–396	10^9/L
Partial thromboplastin time	18.6	10.9–13.6	seconds
Activated partial thromboplastin time	60.5	25.1–33.9	seconds
Fibrinogen	0.25	1.71–3.38	g/L

Blood film: Genuine thrombocytopenia.

47.2.2 BIOCHEMISTRY

	Results	References	Units
Alkaline phosphatase	212	32–93	IU/L
Alanine aminotransferase	133	7–36	IU/L
Lactate dehydrogenase	1824	107–218	IU/L
Total bilirubin	128	4–23	mol/L
Creatinine	336	44.8–80.6	mol/L

47.3 CLINICAL PROGRESS

She was admitted to surgical ward and underwent endoscopic retrograde cholangiopancreatography (ERCP) for deranged liver function. It was normal, but the procedure was complicated by pancreatitis. Bone marrow examination showed reactive marrow with increased iron stain in histiocytes. Haemophagocytosis was occasionally seen (Figure 47.1A). Positron emission tomography/ Computed tomography (PET/CT) showed post-ERCP pancreatitis with peripancreatic oedema and reactive lymph node. There was homogenous fatty infiltration of liver but no specific features of lymphoproliferative disease or malignancy. Spleen and kidneys were normal. Plasma Epstein-Barr virus (EBV) DNA was 673 copies/mL (Normal: Undetectable).

DOI: 10.1201/9781003325413-56

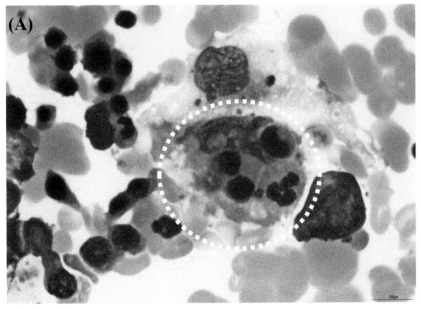

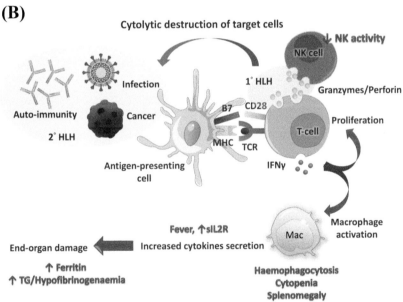

FIGURE 47.1 (A) Bone marrow aspirate showing haemophagocytosis of neutrophil, metamyelocyte, erythroblasts and red cells by histiocytes (dotted circle) (Wright-Giemsa × 1000). (B) Pathogenesis of primary (1°) and secondary (2°) haemophagocytic lymphohistiocytosis (HLH). Diagnostic criteria can be derived from the pathogenesis and are highlighted in red. APC: Antigen-presenting cell; MHC: Major histocompatibility complex; TCR: T-cell receptor; IFNγ: Interferon gamma; NK cell: Natural killer cell; Mac: Macrophage; sIL2R: Soluble interleukin 2 receptor; TG: Triglyceride.

47.4 QUESTIONS

1. What are the possible diagnoses?
2. What are the next investigations?
3. What are the treatment options?

47.5   DIAGNOSIS

The patient's lactate dehydrogenase (LDH) was further increased to a peak of 3530 IU/L. Her ferritin and triglyceride levels were 10901 pmol/L and 35.8 mmol/L, respectively, and blood natural killer (NK) cell cytotoxicity towards K562 cell lines *in vitro*, a measurement of NK cell activities, was reduced. A diagnosis of haemophagocytic lymphohistiocytosis (HLH) was made. She was given a course of corticosteroid, and her fever subsided in 2 days. Ferritin and LDH returned to normal level in 3 weeks.

47.6   PATHOPHYSIOLOGY

HLH is a rare, potentially fatal disorder characterised by dysregulated activation of cytotoxic T-lymphocytes, macrophages or NK cells, increases in circulating cytokine levels and immune-mediated multi-organ injuries. Primary (familial) HLH mostly presents in the first year of life and is caused by inherited gene mutations that perturb cytotoxic T- and NK cell functions, resulting in an immunodeficiency state, hence the inability to clear pathogens. To date, most mutations in primary HLH are related to perforin or defective granule release from cytotoxic T-lymphocytes or NK cells. Genetic defects in inflammasome regulation have also been described. Persistent inflammatory responses increase circulating cytokine levels, and these levels have been shown to upregulate pro-phagocytic signals including calreticulin on mature red cells and downregulate CD47 expression, the "don't eat me signals" on haematopoietic stem cell (HSC). These changes result in increased phagocytosis of HSC and mature red cells. Secondary (acquired) HLH occurs in adults, and unlike primary HLH, its aetiologies are less characterised and likely multifactorial. In fact, some patients with apparent secondary HLH may have inherited gene mutations pertinent to primary HLH. Increased circulating proinflammatory cytokines from macrophages due to sustained toll-like receptor activation, either by infectious agents, autoimmunity or malignancies are the core in pathogenesis. Notable causes associated with secondary HLH include the following. **Infection**: EBV is the most common infectious agent associated with HLH and can occur in both primary and secondary HLH. Patients with COVID-19 infection may also develop cytokine storm similar to that seen in HLH in whom interleukin (IL)-6 has been associated with acute respiratory distress syndrome (ARDS). **Malignancies**: Haematologic malignancies particularly T-cell or NK cell lymphoma are the most common neoplastic cause of HLH. When untreated, it is associated with a rapidly deteriorating course and high mortality. **Rheumatologic**: Rheumatologic cause of HLH is often known as macrophage activation syndrome (MAS). **Iatrogenic**: Haploidentical haematopoietic stem cell transplantation (HSCT), Bi-specific T-cell engager (BiTE), chimeric antigen receptor T-cell therapy and immune checkpoint inhibitors can also result in HLH.

47.7   CLINICAL PRESENTATION

Patients with HLH present with high and persistent fever and a rapidly deteriorating clinical course. Signs and symptoms include fever, jaundice, rash, hepatosplenomegaly, lymphadenopathy, anaemia and bleeding due to coagulopathy and thrombocytopenia. If untreated, patients may develop multi-organ failure. Neurological symptoms are myriad and are associated with serious disease and poor prognosis.

47.8   DIAGNOSIS

Two scoring systems are widely used for the diagnosis of HLH, *viz.*, the revised HLH-2004 criteria (Table 47.1) and the HLH probability calculator (HScore) (http://saintantoine.aphp.fr/score/). These criteria entail identification of genetic mutations and the presence of clinical and laboratory features that are characteristic of HLH (Figure 47.1B).

TABLE 47.1
HLH-2004 Diagnostic Criteria

I. Molecular diagnosis consistent with HLH, or

II. Diagnostic criteria with 5 of 8 of the following symptoms:

1. Fever
2. Splenomegaly
3. Cytopenias affecting > 2 lineages in peripheral blood
   Haemoglobin < 9 g/dL (< 10 g/dL in infants < 4 weeks of age)
   Platelet < 100 × 10^9/L
   Neutrophil < 1 × 10^9/L
4. Fasting triglyceride > 3 mmol/L and/or hypofibrinogenaemia: < 1.5 g/L
5. Haemophagocytosis in the bone marrow, spleen, lymph nodes or liver
6. Low or absent natural killer cell activity
7. Ferritin > 1124 pmol/L
8. Increased soluble CD25 (interleukin-2 receptor) concentration: > 2400 U/mL

47.9 TREATMENT

Patients with HLH show a rapidly progressive clinical course and should receive prompt treatment. In most cases, corticosteroid in the form of dexamethasone is the mainstay of treatment. Subsequent treatment should be individualised. For primary HLH that mostly occurs in paediatric patients, allogeneic HSCT is the curative treatment. For secondary HLH, the underlying causes should be treated. In relapsed or refractory cases, immunosuppressive treatment such as cyclosporin or chemotherapy such as etoposide has been shown to be effective. More recently, monoclonal antibodies targeting IL-1 receptor anakinra, IL-6 receptor tocilizumab, IL-1β canakinumab and tumour necrosis factor (TNF) receptor etanercept have been reported with variable clinical success.

47.10 KEY POINTS

1. HLH is a medical emergency. Patients present acutely with features of multi-organ abnormalities, requiring a high index of suspicion.
2. Primary HLH occurs in infants and is caused by inherited gene mutations that perturb cytotoxic T- and NK cell functions. Secondary HLH occurs in adults, and its aetiologies are diverse.
3. Corticosteroid is the mainstay of treatment and should be given promptly once a diagnosis of HLH has been made. Monoclonal antibodies targeting proinflammatory cytokine signal are emerging.

ADDITIONAL READINGS

1. Ponnatt TS, Lilley CUM, Mirza KM. Hemophagocytic lymphohistiocytosis. Arch Pathol Lab Med 2022; 146: 507–519.
2. Rosee P La, Horne AC, Hines M et al. Recommendations for the management of hemophagocytic lymphohistiocytosis in adults. Blood 2019; 133(23): 2465–2477.
3. Vick EJ, Patel K, Prouet P, Martin MG. Proliferation through activation: hemophagocytic lymphohistiocytosis in hematologic malignancy. Blood Adv 2017; 1(12): 779–791.

48 Hypereosinophilia

48.1 CLINICAL SCENARIO

A 71-year-old woman with good past health presented at the age of 50 with a 6-month history of intermittent vomiting and diarrhoea and was found to have raised absolute eosinophil count (AEC). Stool examination for ova and cysts was negative. Physical examination showed mild eczematous rash over her face and limbs with no lymphadenopathy or hepatosplenomegaly. Upper endoscopy showed gastritis, and biopsy showed only a few scattered eosinophils.

48.2 LABORATORY REPORTS

	Results	References	Units
Haemoglobin	12.4	13.3–17.1	g/dL
White cell count	5.4	3.89–9.93	10^9/L
Platelet count	416	150–400	10^9/L
Eosinophil count	1.5	0.02–0.45	10^9/L
Antinuclear antibody	Negative	Negative	
Antineutrophil cytoplasmic antibody	Negative	Negative	

48.3 QUESTIONS

1. What is the likely diagnosis?
2. What are the differential diagnoses?
3. What is the management plan?

48.4 CLINICAL PROGRESS

Since the initial presentation, the patient has been having occasional diarrhoea and rash with fluctuating eosinophilia for 10 years. Her serum immunoglobulin E was persistently elevated. Ten years later, she was diagnosed with "asthma", requiring intermittent use of inhaled bronchodilators and corticosteroids. Her AEC showed a persistent increase up to 6×10^9/L in 2014 (Figure 48.1A), and the eczematous rash had become more severe, affecting most parts of the body. Bone marrow showed eosinophilia and the presence of eosinophilic myelocytes but no morphological evidence of malignancy (Figure 48.1B). Polymerase chain reaction for T-cell receptor (TCR) showed no clonal rearrangement. Fluorescence in-situ hybridisation (FISH) for *PDGFRA*, *PDGFRB* and *FGFR1* rearrangement was negative. Positron emission tomography/Computed tomography scan showed no evidence of lymphoma. Moreover, she developed severe vomiting and diarrhoea requiring hospital admission. Repeated upper and lower endoscopy showed mild chronic gastritis with scattered eosinophils and colonic polyps with features of adenoma and an increase in eosinophilic infiltrations. She was treated with systemic corticosteroid at 1 mg/kg daily with a resolution of chest and gastrointestinal symptoms and decrease in AEC. However, as the corticosteroid was tapered, her AEC rebounded, and respiratory symptoms recurred. In 2021, she was given mepolizumab, resulting in profound AEC suppression with no recurrence of chest and gastrointestinal symptoms nearly 2 years since commencement of treatment (Figure 48.1C).

DOI: 10.1201/9781003325413-57

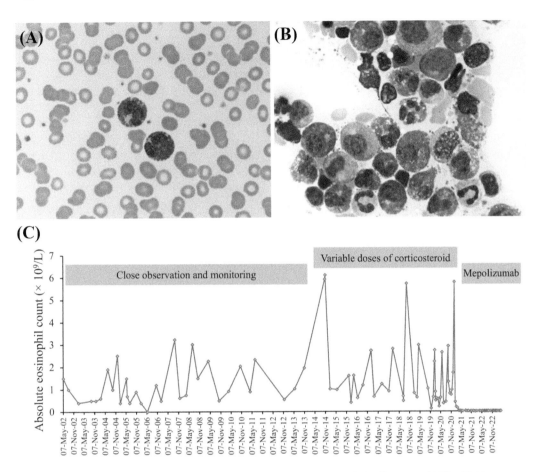

FIGURE 48.1 (A) Peripheral blood smear showing eosinophilia (Wright-Giemsa × 1000). (B) Bone marrow aspirate showing increased eosinophils and eosinophilic myelocytes to 35%, left-shifted granulopoiesis and depressed erythroid activity (Wright-Giemsa × 1000). (C) Haematological response to corticosteroid and interleukin-5 monoclonal antibody mepolizumb.

48.5 EOSINOPHILIA

For most laboratories, the upper limit of normal eosinophil count is $0.5 \times 10^9/L$. Eosinophilia is defined by an AEC $> 0.5 \times 10^9/L$, whereas hypereosinophilia (HE) is defined by AEC $> 1.5 \times 10^9/L$. In the investigation of eosinophilia, **reactive causes** should be considered including tissue-invasive parasitic infestations, allergy or atopic conditions, collagen vascular disease, particularly eosinophilic granulomatosis with polyangiitis (EGPA or Churg-Strauss syndrome), granulomatosis with polyangiitis (Wegener's granulomatosis), pulmonary eosinophilic diseases such as idiopathic acute or chronic eosinophilic pneumonia and allergic bronchopulmonary aspergillosis (ABPA), allergic gastroenteritis and endocrine disorders such as adrenal insufficiency.

In contrast, **lymphoproliferative diseases** may result in secondary eosinophilia due to production of cytokines from neoplastic lymphoid cells, particularly T-cell lymphoma and Hodgkin lymphoma and acute lymphoblastic leukaemia. Eosinophilia may also result from **primary bone marrow disorder**. In particular, myeloid/lymphoid neoplasms with eosinophilia encompass a group of diseases characterised by *FIP1L1::PDGFRA* fusion and other translocations involving *PDGFRB*, *FGFR1* and *JAK2* detectable by FISH and karyotyping. WHO-defined myeloid neoplasms including myelodysplasic syndrome (MDS), myeloproliferative neoplasm (MPN), MDS/ MPN, systemic mastocytosis and acute myeloid leukemia may also be associated with eosinophilia, but they are diagnosed by their characteristic haematological changes. A negative screen for these disorders should prompt the consideration of chronic eosinophilic leukaemia (CEL), characterised by the presence of dysplasia in different lineages, an increase in blasts (< 20% in blood and bone marrow) and clonal haematopoiesis. In addition, a subgroup of patients with unexplained eosino- philia may show evidence of underlying clonal T-cells with aberrant immunophenotypes, known as **lymphocyte-variant HE**. The size of an abnormal T-cell clone is small, and lymphocyte count is usually normal. This is distinct from the secondary cause of eosinophilia due to T-cell lymphoma in which clinical disease is apparent. Patients without evidence of these primary diseases will be diagnosed with **idiopathic** HE and those with end organ damage will be diagnosed with idiopathic hypereosinophilic syndrome (HES).

48.6   HYPEREOSINOPHILIC SYNDROME

Conventionally, HES was defined as idiopathic HE for at least 6 months with evidence of organ infil- tration. More recently, the definition has been broadened to include other known association with HE, and diagnosis is made based on AEC > 1.5×10^9/L on 2 examinations at least 1 month apart with evidence of end organ dysfunction attributable to the eosinophilia, irrespective of the cause. With this new definition, HES includes (1) myeloid HE/HES, (2) lymphocytic variant HE/HES, (3) overlap HES (eosinophilic gastrointestinal disorders and eosinophilic granulomatosis with polyangiitis), (4) associated HE/HES (in the context of a defined disorder including parasitic infestation, lymphoma, immunodeficiency or hypersensitivity reaction), (5) familial HE/HES (> 1 family member excluding associated HE/HES) and (6) idiopathic HE/HES (unknown cause and exclusion of other subtypes).

48.7   CLINICAL PRESENTATION

Clinical presentation reflects the extent and severity of organ involvement. No organ is spared although skin, lungs, gastrointestinal tract and the heart are frequently involved. Common derma- tological presentations include generalised pruritus, urticaria or eczema. Pulmonary manifesta- tions include asthma, pulmonary fibrosis or radiological evidence of pulmonary infiltrates. Cardiac involvement can lead to severe consequences including endomyocardial fibrosis, intracardiac thrombi (also known as Löffler's endocarditis), thromboembolic complications, perimyocarditis, pericardial effusion and heart failure. Gastrointestinal involvement includes oesophagitis, gastroen- teritis and serositis. As some of these clinical conditions themselves can give rise to eosinophilia, definitive diagnosis may sometimes be difficult (see the following).

48.8   MANAGEMENT

Patients with eosinophilia should be investigated to **identify secondary causes** that can be modi- fied or eradicated. This entails a complete drug, allergy and travel history and enquiry of respira- tory, bowel, musculoskeletal and constitutional symptoms. Physical signs related to specific causes include rash, signs of respiratory and cardiovascular diseases, lymphadenopathy or organomegaly. Subsequent investigations should be guided by the clinical suspicion. Patients without apparent secondary causes should be investigated for **primary blood disorders** that are associated with eosinophilia. The investigation entails examination of blood smear and bone marrow, cytogenetic analyses and next generation sequencing to identify underlying clonal disorder. Flow cytometry and T-cell receptor rearrangement tests should be considered even in the absence of lymphocy- tosis to identify small T-cell clone underlying lymphocyte-variant HE. The extent and severity of organ involvement in idiopathic HES should be investigated, even in asymptomatic patients. This entails chest X-ray, CT thorax for pulmonary infiltrate, blood tests for pro B-type natriuretic peptide (proBNP) and troponin I (TnI), echocardiography and cardiac magnetic resonance imaging for cardiac involvement. In patients with dermatological or gastrointestinal tract manifestations, biopsies are warranted to investigate tissue infiltrations.

First-line treatment of idiopathic HES is oral corticosteroid at 1 mg/kg prednisolone or equivalent, with dose adjustment based on clinical conditions. Decrease in AEC is usually rapid, and thereafter, the steroid dose should be gradually tapered to avoid side effects. Patients with steroid-dependent eosinophilia should be given steroid sparing agents, including methotrexate, mycophenolate mofetil or cyclophosphamide. In refractory cases, antagonist of interleukin (IL)-5, which is the key mediator of eosinophilia, should be considered. Monoclonal anti-IL-5 antibody mepolizumab was recently approved for this indication, and other monoclonal antibodies against IL-5 and IL-5 receptor are under investigation. The potential effects of long-term suppression of eosinophils are currently unclear.

48.9 KEY POINTS

1. Idiopathic HES is a diagnosis by exclusion. Reactive causes and primary blood disorders associated with eosinophilia should be excluded.
2. Organ infiltration by eosinophilia is the main cause of morbidity. Skin, lungs, gastrointestinal tract and the heart are the main organs affected.
3. In addition to corticosteroid, antagonists of IL-5, a key mediator of eosinophilia, are now available for treatment.

ADDITIONAL READINGS

1. Klion AD. Approach to the patient with suspected hypereosinophilic syndrome. Hematology Am Soc Hematol Educ Program 2022; 2022(1): 47–54.
2. Shomali W, Gotlib J. World health organization-defined eosinophilic disorders: 2022 update on diagnosis, risk stratification, and management. Am J Hematol 2022; 97: 129–148.
3. Schwaab J, Lübke J, Reiter A, Metzgeroth G. Idiopathic hypereosinophilic syndrome-diagnosis and treatment. Allergo J Int 2022; 31: 251–256.

49 IgG4–Related Disease

49.1 CLINICAL SCENARIO

A 58-year-old woman with a 10-year history of rheumatoid arthritis (RA) presented with fever and abdominal pain. Physical examination showed non-tender enlargement of the right submandibular gland and a right groin lymph node, both about 2 cm in size. She was taking 5 mg prednisolone daily for her RA. Previous treatment with weekly methotrexate, which she had received for the past 5 years, was stopped a few months ago. Positron emission tomography/Computed tomography (PET/CT) scan showed enlargement and increased metabolic activity of the right submandibular gland and multiple cervical, axillary and groin lymph nodes.

Submandibulectomy was performed. The salivary gland was infiltrated by lymphoid cells forming reactive lymphoid follicles. Plasma cells were present, and the immunoglobulin (Ig) G4/IgG ratio was 50%. The plasma cells were polytypic for kappa and lambda light chains (Figures 49.1A and 49.1B). There was minimal fibrosis in the salivary gland. There was no demonstrable immunoglobulin heavy chain (IgH) and T-cell receptor (TCR) rearrangement.

49.2 LABORATORY REPORTS

	Results	References	Units
C-reactive protein	< 0.35	< 0.76	mg/dL
Immunoglobulin A	213	70–386	mg/dL
Immunoglobulin G	5525	819–1725	mg/dL
Immunoglobulin M	95	55–307	mg/dL
Immunoglobulin G4	34.5	0.09–1.46	g/L

Serum protein electrophoresis showed no monoclonal band. Complement C3, C4 levels were normal.

49.3 QUESTIONS

1. What is the likely diagnosis?
2. What are the next investigations?
3. What is the principle of management?

49.4 IGG4–RELATED DISEASE

The patient was diagnosed immunoglobulin G4–related disease (IgG4–RD). IgG4–RD is a chronic immune-mediated disease with protean manifestations including parotid and submandibular salivary gland and lacrimal gland enlargement, lymphadenopathy, orbital pseudotumour, pancreatitis, sclerosing cholangitis, retroperitoneal fibrosis and tubulointerstitial nephritis, which may occur simultaneously or in a metachronous fashion. There is a 2:1 male preponderance, and the median age at diagnosis is 60–70 years. **Diagnosis can be made on histological and serological grounds after exclusion of differential diagnoses.** Histological features are characterised by the presence of i) a dense lymphoplasmacytic infiltrate enriched with IgG4 positive plasma cells; ii) storiform fibrosis characterised by a swirling, "cartwheel" pattern of fibrosis; and iii) obliterative phlebitis in which venous channels are obliterated by an inflammatory lymphoplasmacytic infiltrate. As a

DOI: 10.1201/9781003325413-58

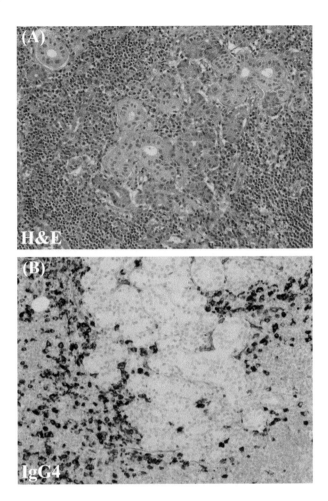

FIGURE 49.1   (A) H&E section showing dense infiltration of the submandibular gland by lymphocytes and plasma cells. (B) The infiltrate was positive for immunoglobulin G4. (*Figures 49.1A and 49.1B, courtesy of Dr. Rex Au Yeung.*)

diagnostic prerequisite, the IgG4:IgG plasma cell ratio has to be greater than 40%. Serum IgG4 levels are elevated in approximately 70% of cases. Although mildly increased serum IgG4 (1.5–5 g/L) is non-specific, a markedly elevated level (> 5 g/L) is virtually specific for IgG4–RD. Eosinophilia and polyclonal hypergammaglobulinaemia are associated features in IgG4–RD and may pose diagnostic challenges. The pathogenesis of IgG4–RD is presently unclear, although CD4+SLAMF7+ cytotoxic T-lymphocytes, which produce profibrotic and inflammatory cytokines such as interleukin-1, transforming growth factor-β, interferon γ and cytolytic molecules may play a pathogenic role. These cytotoxic T-lymphocytes may be activated by the continuous antigen presentation by B-cells and plasmablasts, which produce IgG4 and IgE.

49.5   INVESTIGATIONS

In addition to the tissue biopsy and serum level of IgG4, investigations should be performed to exclude alternative diagnoses and evaluate the extent of disease. Serum protein electrophoresis and IgG subclass evaluation should be performed to rule out monoclonal gammopathy. The urine albumin/creatinine ratio and serum C3 and C4 levels should be examined to assess for renal involvement. PET/CT is also advisable. Renal biopsy is indicated in patients with proteinuria or renal lesions on imaging. Two distinct histological patterns have been reported, namely, hypocomplementaemic tubulointerstitial nephritis in 80% of cases, and membranoproliferative glomerulonephritis in 20% of cases. Bone marrow examination is of relatively low diagnostic value.

49.6   DIFFERENTIAL DIAGNOSES

Diagnostic challenges of IgG4–RD arise from its protean clinical presentations and the fact that neither the presence of IgG4-positive plasma cells in tissues nor an increase in serum IgG4 is specific for IgG4–RD. Moreover, eosinophilia and polyclonal hypergammaglobulinaemia can occur in other various medical conditions other than IgG4–RD. Differential diagnoses of IgG–RD include multicentric Castleman disease, histiocytic disorders, e.g., Rosai–Dorfman disease or Erdheim–Chester disease, extra-pulmonary sarcoidosis, lymphoma particularly mucosal associated lymphoid tissue (MALT) lymphoma of the salivary and lacrimal glands, hypereosinophilic syndrome and multiple myeloma. Early diagnosis is essential for this treatable condition and to avoid potentially lethal fibrotic disease, particularly retroperitoneal fibrosis, periaortitis, coronary arteritis and late complications such as chronic pancreatitis, which can be irreversible.

49.7   TREATMENT

Corticosteroids are the first-line therapy for most patients, with an overall response rate > 90%. Rituximab has also been shown to be highly effective with a response rate of 97%. For refractory cases, anecdotal reports showed that chemoimmunotherapy as used in lymphoma may be effective. Theoretically, elotuzumab targeting the pathogenic CD4+ SLAMF7+ cytotoxic T-lymphocytes and anti-IgE therapy with omalizumab are potentially useful, but their therapeutic roles in IgG4–RD remain to be determined.

49.8   KEY POINTS

1. IgG4–RD is a chronic immune-mediated disease with protean manifestations.
2. Diagnosis is based on histological and serological grounds after exclusion of differential diagnoses.
3. Corticosteroid and rituximab are the mainstays of treatment.

ADDITIONAL READING

1. Chen LYC, Mattman A, Seidman MA, Carruthers MN. IgG4-related disease: what a hematologist needs to know. Haematologica 2019; 104(3): 444–455.

50 Lymphadenopathy and Hypergammaglobulinaemia

50.1 CLINICAL SCENARIO

A 58-year-old retired businessman with good past health presented with subjective weight loss of 5 kg since April 2021. He was otherwise well. He was married, and his wife and two daughters were staying abroad. Family history was unremarkable. Physical examination showed generalised lymphadenopathy in the neck, axillae and groins. Positron emission tomography/Computed tomography confirmed multiple lymph nodes of low SUVmax (Figure 50.1). Excision biopsy of the right groin lymph node showed follicular hyperplasia consistent with reactive changes and no evidence of lymphoma.

50.2 LABORATORY REPORTS

	Results	References	Unit
Haemoglobin	13.2	13–17	g/dL
White cell count	4.7	4–10	10^9/L
Platelet count	191	150–400	10^9/L
Globulin	64	24–26	g/L
Immunoglobulin G/A/M	3360/1200/351	1560/453/304 (ULN)	mg/dL
M-Protein	Absent	Absent	
Erythrocyte sedimentation rate	72	< 20	mm/hr

ULN: Upper limit of normal. Blood smear showed normal differential count. Liver and renal function: Normal.

50.3 QUESTIONS

1. What are the possible causes of his condition?
2. What additional information is needed from the patient?
3. What further investigations should be performed?

50.4 CAUSES

Generalised lymphadenopathy is defined by the abnormal enlargement of more than two non-contiguous lymph node groups. There are a number of causes.

1. Lymphoproliferative diseases including lymphoma are a common cause. Generalised lymphadenopathy can also occur in acute lymphoblastic leukaemia and occasionally, in acute myeloid leukaemia. A specific subtype of T-cell lymphoma, known as **angio-immunoblastic T-cell lymphoma**, is characteristically associated with polyclonal hypergammaglobulinaemia.
2. Infections, particularly systemic viral infections such as infectious mononucleosis due to primary infection with Epstein–Barr Virus or cytomegalovirus, are another cause.

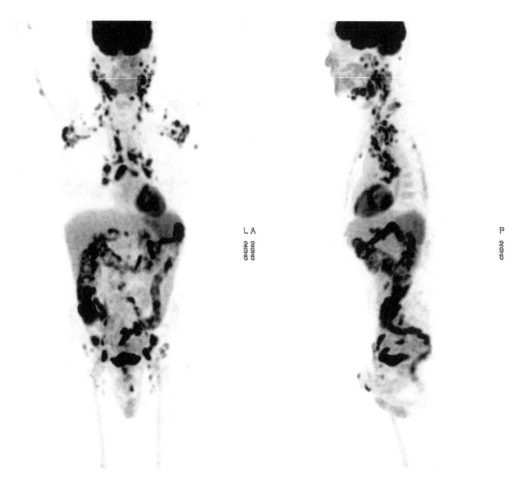

FIGURE 50.1   Positron emission tomography/Computed tomography scan of the patient showing gener-alised lymphadenopathy in the neck, axillae, mediastinum, abdomen and groin after human immunodefi-ciency virus infection.

These infections are associated with rash, fever, hepatitis and atypical lymphocytosis. Hepatosplenomegaly, which is typically mild, may be present. **Human immunodeficiency virus (HIV)** infection is associated with generalised lymphadenopathy and polyclonal hypergammaglobulinaemia. Other examples of infective causes of generalised lymphade-nopathy include *mycobacterium tuberculosis*, typhoid fever caused by *Salmonella* Typhi and rickettsial diseases.

3. Autoimmune and inflammatory diseases can cause generalised lymphadenopathy and hypergammaglobulinaemia. In particular, **multicentric Castleman disease and IgG4–related diseases** are defined by their characteristic histological and immunohistochemical features and are associated with hypergammaglobulinaemia.

4. A number of drugs are known to be associated with generalised lymphadenopathy, includ-ing phenytoin and penicillamine. This usually occurs within a few weeks after intake of incriminating agents and can be associated with maculopapular rash, fever, hepato-splenomegaly and liver function abnormalities. The symptoms usually resolve within a few months after cessation of drug intake.

50.5   INVESTIGATIONS

Investigations should aim at differentiating neoplastic from reactive causes. For patients with generalised lymphadenopathy of a significant size, excisional biopsy rather than core biopsy or fine needle aspiration is recommended to ensure adequate tissues for a complete histological examination and immunohistochemical investigation. For reactive causes of generalised lymphadenopathy, microbiology, immunology and serology tests should be performed and interpreted with clinical data.

50.6   CLINICAL PROGRESS

Virologic workup revealed HIV-1/-2 antibody positive, which was confirmed by Western blot. The patient volunteered that he had unprotected sexual activities with multiple male partners. A diagnosis of generalised lymphadenopathy due to HIV infection was made.

50.7   HUMAN IMMUNODEFICIENCY VIRUS (HIV) INFECTION

Upon acquisition of HIV, the virus primarily infects CD4+ T-cells and spreads to the lymphoid organs within days. The virus then enters the bloodstream and multiplies exponentially in the next few weeks, reaching a peak on approximately day 30, when HIV antibody become detectable. Clinical manifestations, known as acute retroviral syndrome, are variable, but they include fever, generalised lymphadenopathy, rash, myalgia and malaise. Thereafter, immune response develops, and HIV load decreases to a steady state known as the "setpoint" when HIV replication becomes relatively stable, often for years. The levels of "setpoint" show wide variation in different patients. If untreated, then HIV causes progressive loss of CD4+ T-cells and immunological abnormalities, resulting in immunodeficiency, opportunistic infections and oncogenesis. During the course of the disease, HIV infection is associated with hypergammaglobulinaemia due to activation of naïve B-cells as the result of direct viral infection, increased cytokines or abnormal helper regulation.

50.8   KEY POINTS

1. Generalised lymphadenopathy can be due to neoplastic, infective, immune/inflammatory and drug causes.
2. Generalised lymphadenopathy can occur early in the course of HIV infection and is associated with hypergammaglobulinaemia.

ADDITIONAL READING

1. Deeks SG, Overbaugh J, Philips A, Buchbinder S. HIV infection. Nat Rev Dis Primers 2015; 1: 15035.

51 Paraneoplastic Pemphigus

51.1 CLINICAL SCENARIO

A 58-year-old man with good past health presented with balanitis in September 2020, followed 2 months later by progressive oral ulcers. He was initially treated by private practitioner with a course of antibiotics and corticosteroids without significant improvement. Physical examination (Figures 51.1A and 51.1B) showed generalised erosive mucosal lesions in the oral cavity with easy desquamation, exposing raw surface underneath. His lips were swollen, and there was trismus due to pain. There was generalised maculopapular rash, blisters on legs and a vaguely palpable central abdominal mass. He had been a chronic smoker but quit more than 10 years ago.

51.2 LABORATORY REPORTS

	Results	References	Unit
C-reactive protein	4.2	< 0.76	mg/dL
Anti-nuclear antibody	1/320	< 1/80	
Anti-skin antibody	1/640	Negative	

Complete blood count was unremarkable. Serum albumin was 32 g/L; otherwise, kidney and liver functions were normal.

Oral mucosal biopsy showed only ulceration, and skin biopsy revealed subepidermal blistering. Positron emission tomography/Computed tomography (PET/CT) scan showed hypermetabolic retroperitoneal soft tissue mass in abdomen and multiple peripancreatic, para-aortic lymphadenopathy and bilateral cervical lymphadenopathy (Figures 51.1C and 51.1D). Other organs, including the lungs, were unremarkable. CT-guided biopsy of the retroperitoneal lymph node showed follicular lymphoma grade 1. The patient was otherwise well and could climb 3 flights of stairs.

51.3 QUESTIONS

1. What is the dermatological diagnosis?
2. What is the overall clinical condition?
3. What is the prognosis of this patient?

51.4 CLINICAL PROGRESS

A diagnosis of paraneoplastic pemphigus (PNP) was made. The patient received a combination of obinutuzumab and bendamustine (OB) for the treatment of lymphoma. After 3 courses, oral mucositis and balanitis partially improved, but the rash was persistent. Interim PET/CT scan showed residual soft tissue in the abdomen. Thereafter, he presented with fever and shortness of breath, and the sputum grew methicillin-sensitive *Staphylococcus aureus*. Despite adequate response to intravenous antibiotics and the resolution of pneumonia, he became progressively short-of-breath, requiring oxygen support most of the day. A spirometry was performed, showing FEV1 2.63 litres, FEV1/FVC 59%, FEF25–75% 0.92 L/sec (20% expected) and normal FVC.

DOI: 10.1201/9781003325413-60

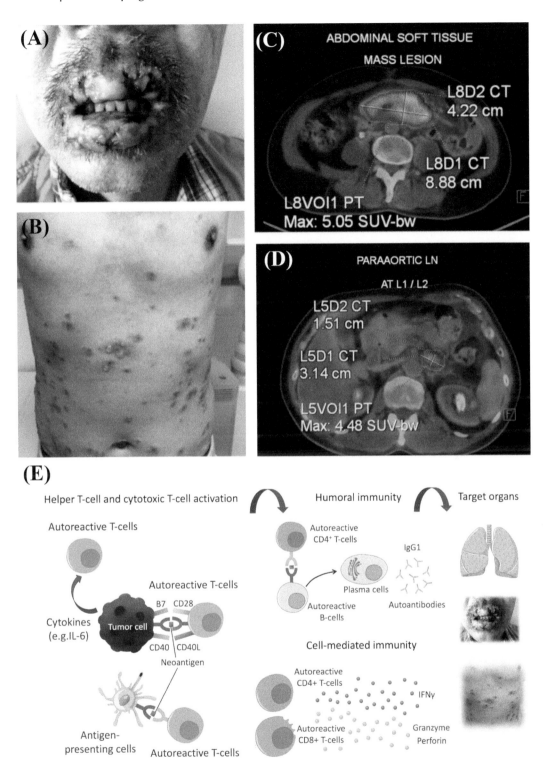

FIGURE 51.1 Clinical features of a paraneoplastic pemphigus (PNP) patient. (A) Erosive mucosal lesions affecting the buccal mucosa and lips. (B) Generalised maculopapular rash some of which formed blisters. Positron emission tomography/Computed tomography scan showing (C) central abdominal mass and (D) paraaortic lymph nodes. (E) Pathogenesis of PNP. IL: Interleukin; IFNγ: Interferon gamma.

51.5   PARANEOPLASTIC PEMPHIGUS

PNP is an autoimmune, blistering skin diseases associated with underlying malignancy. It was first described 30 years ago and is characterised by **clinical manifestations** of painful and progressive stomatitis and blistering and erosive skin lesions; **serological evidence** of autoantibodies against antigens in the desmosomes (connection between keratinocytes), most frequently the plakin family proteins and hemidesmosomes (connections between epidermis and dermis); **histological evidence** of acantholysis, lichenoid or interface dermatitis; and the presence of an **underlying malignancy**. The latter is most frequently haematological, with non-Hodgkin lymphoma, chronic lymphocytic leukaemia and Castleman disease being the most common associations.

Clinically, stomatitis, characterised by erosion and ulceration of the oropharynx, is the first presenting symptoms in most patients and may persist throughout the course of the disease. Other mucosal surfaces including the genital tract may also be affected. Dermatological manifestations are variable within the same patient and among different patients. Blisters and erosions are most common, reminiscent of pemphigus vulgaris, bullous pemphigoid, erythema multiforme or toxic epidermal necrolysis. Erythematous papules and plagues similar to lichen planus may also develop. About 30% of patients develop bronchiolitis obliterans (BO), presenting with progressive dyspnoea. This is associated with inferior treatment outcomes and prognosis and is a common cause of mortality in these patients.

51.6   PATHOGENESIS

A number of pathogenetic pathways that link the underlying malignancies and the mucocutaneous and pulmonary manifestations have been proposed (Figure 51.1E). Specifically, **neoplastic cells can activate both CD4+ helper T-cells and CD8+ cytotoxic T-cells** via antigen presentation either directly by themselves or indirectly by professional antigen-presenting cells. They can also secrete cytokines, e.g., interleukin (IL)-6 that is thought to suppress regulatory T-cells and drive them into effector T-cells. Humoral and cell-mediated autoimmunity are involved. The autoreactive helper T-cells activate and differentiate B-cells into plasma cells that produce the autoantibodies. The autoreactive helper and cytotoxic T-cells can also produce interferon γ, granzyme and perforin. Activation of autoimmunity results in end organ injury characteristic of PNP. Mechanisms underlying the preferential damage of mucocutaneous and pulmonary tissues are unclear. It is possible that the T-cell response to tumour antigen can cross-react with self-antigens from these tissues, thereby causing autoimmunity due to molecular mimicry.

51.7   TREATMENT

The rarity of PNP has precluded large-scale clinical trials, and recommendations are based on anecdotes and small patient cohorts. In principle, treatment should focus on management of the mucocutaneous lesions, underlying malignancies and BO. Systemic corticosteroids are the mainstays of treatment. For patients with severe mucosal lesions, cyclosporin or dexamethasone mouthwash can be given. Symptomatic control for painful stomatitis is important. Intravenous immunoglobulin, plasmapheresis and anti-CD20 therapy have also been used. Treatment of underlying lymphoproliferative diseases should begin as soon as patients can tolerate it, but not infrequently, the mucocutaneous and pulmonary diseases may persist despite reduction of the tumour load. Treatment of lymphoma has immunosuppressive effects that may also serve to dampen the autoreactive immune response. More specifically, Bruton's tyrosine kinase inhibitor ibrutinib disrupts B-cell signaling and hence may reduce the production of autoantibodies, which are core to the pathogenesis of PNP. However, tocilizumab and siltuximab, monoclonal antibodies used against IL-6 receptors and IL-6 itself that are effective for Castleman disease, may also help to ameliorate the active IL-6 signaling that is of pathogenetic significance in PNP. Management of

BO is challenging, and inhaled bronchodilators, corticosteroids and immunomodulatory agents are often used but with uncertain benefits. In fact, progressive BO with respiratory failure is a major cause of mortality in these patients.

51.8   KEY POINTS

1. There is a clinical triad of PNP, BO and underlying haematological malignancies.
2. Underlying malignancies may trigger humoral and cellular immunities, leading to end organ damage involving mucocutaneous and pulmonary tissues.
3. Outcome is dismal, and mortality can be related to respiratory complications.

ADDITIONAL READINGS

1. Kim JH, Kim SC. Paraneoplastic pemphigus: paraneoplastic autoimmune disease of the skin and mucosa. Front Immunol 2019; 10: 1–11.
2. Ouedraogo E, Gottlieb J, de Masson A et al. Risk factors for death and survival in paraneoplastic pemphigus associated with hematologic malignancies in adults. J Am Cad Dermatol 2019; 80(6): 1544–1549.
3. Anhalt GJ, Kim S, Stanley JR et al. Paraneoplastic pemphigus: an autoimmune mucocutaneous disease associated with neoplasia. N Engl J Med 1990; 323(25): 1729–1735.

Index

Note: Page numbers in *italics* indicate a figure and page numbers in **bold** indicate a table on the corresponding page.

A

acquired Factor VIII inhibitor
    APTT, *15*
    causes of, 16
    clinical progress, 14
    clinical scenario, 14
    definitive tests, 16
    easy bruising, 14
    isolated APTT prolongation, 14–16
    laboratory confirmation of, 16
    laboratory reports, 14
    questions, 14
    treatment, 16–17
acquired Factor V inhibitor
    APTT, 18–19
    clinical presentation, 19
    clinical progress, 18
    clinical scenario, 18
    coagulation pathway, *19*
    hypertension and hypertensive nephropathy, 18
    laboratory abnormalities, 19–20
    laboratory reports, 18
    management, 20
    PT, 18–19
    questions, 18
acquired haemophilia, *see* acquired Factor VIII inhibitor
activated partial thromboplastin time (APTT), *see also* isolated APTT prolongation
    in acquired Factor VIII inhibitor, *15*
    in acquired Factor V (FV) inhibitor, 18–19
    TTP, 173
activated prothrombin complex concentrate (aPCC), 9, *15*, 20
acute chest syndrome, 129
acute kidney injury, 178–179
acute myeloid leukaemia I (AML)
    bone marrow aspirate, *32*
    clinical presentation, 33
    clinical progress, 31–32
    clinical scenario, 31
    diagnosis, 32–33
    easy bruising, 31
    genetic analysis, 23
    laboratory reports, 31
    management of, 33–34
    MRD monitoring, 33
    prognostication, 33
    questions, 31
    shortness of breath, 31
acute myeloid leukaemia II (AML)
    BCL2 inhibitor, 37
    blood film, *36*
    clinical scenario, 35
    definition, 35–37
    diabetes mellitus, 35
    hyperlipidaemia, 35
    laboratory reports, 35
    patient progress, 35
    questions, 35
    treatment, 37
acute sickling crises, 129–130
adenosine diphosphate (ADP), 187
adriamycin, bleomycin, vinblastine and darcarbazine (ABVD), 98
AIHA, *see* autoimmune haemolytic anaemia (AIHA)
amyloid A (AA) amyloidosis, 105
amyloid light chain (AL) amyloidosis, 105
amyloidosis
    clinical presentation, 105
    clinical scenario, 103
    definition, 105
    diagnosis, 103–104
    hyperlipidaemia, 103
    hypertension, 103
    investigations, 105–106
    laboratory reports, 103
    light microscopy, *104*
    management, 106
    questions, 103
amyloid transthyretin (ATTR) amyloidosis, 105
anaemia exacerbation, 129
angioimmunoblastic T-cell lymphoma, 207
angiotensin converting enzyme inhibitor (ACEI), 106
angiotensin renin blocker (ARB), 106
anti-platelet autoantibody, 184
aplastic anaemia (AA)
    clinical progress, 138
    clinical scenario, 137
    definition, 139
    differential diagnosis, 139
    haematological response, *138*
    investigations, 137
    laboratory reports, 137
    management, 140
    menstruation, 137
    pathophysiology, 139
    questions, 137
APTT, *see* activated partial thromboplastin time (APTT)
asthma, 61
atypical haemolytic uraemic syndrome (aHUS), 175
    α thalassaemia, 177
    classification, 179
    clinical progress, 178
    clinical scenario, 177
    definition, 178–179
    diagnosis, 179
    laboratory reports, 177
    management, 179
    microangiopathic haemolytic anaemia, *178*
    questions, 177–178
    thrombocytopenia, *178*
    thrombotic microangiopathy, 178
autoimmune haemolytic anaemia (AIHA), 153, 156

autoimmunity, 147
autologous HSCT, 111
avascular necrosis, 130

B

BCL2 inhibitor, 37
beta-2 microglobulin amyloidosis, 105
beta (β) thalassaemia
    clinical features, 121
    clinical progress, 119
    clinical scenario, 119
    clinicopathologic changes, 121
    complications, 121–122
    diagnosis, 121
    facial features of patient, *120*
    genetic modifiers, 120–121
    genetics, 120
    laboratory reports, 119
    management, 122
    questions, 119
    transfusion-dependent thalassaemia, 119
biliary pancreatitis, 159
biliary stones, 130
Bing Neel syndrome, 72
bi-nucleated Reed Sternberg cells, 96
bleeding
    acquired Factor V inhibitor, 18
    AML, 33
    amyloidosis, 105
    CML, 44
    diathesis, 22
    DIC, 22
    DLBCL, 69
    ET, 50
    Factor VII deficiency, 11
    hereditary macrothrombocytopenia, 187
    HLH, 198
    IDA, 143
    isolated APTT prolongation, 16
    ITP, 185
    multiple myeloma, 110
    myeloid neoplasm with germline predisposition, 60
    NK/T-cell lymphoma, 87
    PMF, 54
    severe haemophilia, 7
    tendency, 72
    TTP, 173
    VTE, 27
    VWD, 3
    WM, 72
blood
    abnormal tests, 11
    AIHA, 153
    CAD, 156
    cancer, 58
    CD, 193
    count, 5, 24, 40
    deletional HbH disease, *124*
    disease/malignancies, 31, 48
    donors/recombinant products, 9
    film, 35, **36**, 83
    G6PD deficiency, 159
    GPI, 138

    hairy cells, *81*
    hereditary macrothrombocytopenia, 187
    HLH, 196
    HS, 163
    HUS, 178
    hypereosinophilia, 202
    ITP, 183
    loss in genital tract, 143
    lymphoma cells, 88
    PaO_2 in, 131
    parameters, 39
    paravalvular leak, 166
    PNH, 169
    PNP, 210
    SCD, 129
    smear, *44*, *49*, *52*, 55
    T-PLL cells, *94*
    transfusions, 19, 54
    TTP, 173
    turbulent flow, 22
    vitamin B12 deficiency anaemia, 145
bone marrow failure (BMF), 137
brain natriuretic peptide (BNP), 106
Bruton's tyrosine kinase (BTK), 78

C

caplacizumab, 176
cardiac prosthesis-related haemolytic anaemia, 167
Castleman disease (CD)
    clinical progress, 193
    clinical scenario, 193
    definition, 193–195
    diagnosis, 195
    laboratory reports, 193
    lymph node, *194*
    malaise, 193
    management, 195
    questions, 193
cell of origin (COO), 69
central nervous system (CNS), 62
chimeric antigen receptor T-cell (CART) therapy, 111
chronic inflammatory demyelinating
    polyradiculoneuropathy (CIDP), 115
chronic lymphocytic leukaemia (CLL)
    Binet staging system, **78**
    blood smear of, *76*
    clinical progress, 75–76
    clinical scenario, 75
    definition, 77
    diagnosis, 77
    IPI scoring system, **78**
    laboratory reports, 75
    lymphadenopathy, 75
    prognostication, 77–78
    questions, 75
    Rai staging system, **77**
chronic myeloid leukaemia (CML)
    clinical presentation, 44
    clinical progress, 43
    clinical scenario, 43
    coronary artery disease, 43
    laboratory diagnosis, 46
    laboratory reports, 43

management, 46
natural disease course, 46
pathogenesis, 43–44
percutaneous coronary intervention, 43
peripheral blood smear, *44*
prognostic factors, 46
questions, 43
TKI, 46–47
chronic myeloid leukaemia in the chronic phase
        (CML-CP), 43
chronic red cell transfusion, 121
chronic sickle cell diseases, 130
classical Hodgkin lymphoma (cHL), 96
classical Hodgkin lymphoma, nodular sclerosing type
        (cHL-NS), 96, *97*
cold agglutinin disease (CAD)
        clinical progress, 156
        clinical scenario, 156
        definition, 156–157, 158
        haemoglobin levels, *157*
        haemolysis in, 157–158
        investigations, 158
        laboratory reports, 156
        questions, 156
        retroperitoneal leiomyosarcoma, 156
        treatment, 158
computed tomography (CT), 24
continuous ambulatory peritoneal dialysis
        (CAPD), 187
coronary artery disease, 43
corticosteroid, 176, 185, 206
crizanlizumab, 129
cryoglobulinaemia, 72
cutaneous T-cell lymphoma (CTCL), 90
cytogenetic analysis, 55
cytopenia of undetermined significance (CCUS), 41

D

deep vein thrombosis (DVT), 24
deoxyhaemoglobin (deoxyHb), 132
diepoxybutane (DEB), 137
diffuse large B-cell lymphoma (DLBCL)
        aetiology, 67
        cell of origin, 69
        clinical presentation, 69
        clinical scenario, 67
        definition, 67
        management, 69–70
        molecular landscape, 69
        not otherwise specified (NOS), 67
        PET/CT, *68*
        prognostication, 70
direct antiglobulin test (DAT), 153, 176
direct oral anticoagulant (DOAC), 14, 27
disseminated intravascular coagulopathy (DIC)
        clinical scenario, 21
        diagnosis, 21–22
        hypertension, 21
        laboratory reports, 21
        management, 23
        pathogenesis, 22
        pathogenesis of, *22*
        questions, 21

E

easy bruising
        AA, 137
        acquired haemophilia, 14
        AML, 31
        ITP, 183
        PNH, 169
        VWF, 1
eczema, 96
endoscopic retrograde cholangiopancreatography
        (ERCP), 196
endothelial damage, 179
eosin-5-maleimide (EMA), 164
eosinophilia, 201–202
Epstein–Barr virus (EBV) infection, 87, 198
erythematous rash, *see* mycosis fungoides (MF)
erythroblasts, 141
essential thrombocytosis (ET)
        clinical presentation, 48–49
        clinical progress, 48
        clinical scenario, 48
        complications, 50
        differential diagnosis, 48–49
        genetics, 49–50
        laboratory reports, 48
        prognosis, 50
        questions, 48
        treatment, 50
extracorporeal photopheresis (ECP), 92

F

Factor VII deficiency
        carcinoma, 11
        clinical penetrance, 12
        clinical scenario, 11
        definition, 12
        differential diagnosis, 13
        laboratory reports, 11
        physiological function of, *12*
        progress, 11
        questions, 11
        treatment, 13
        vitamin K-dependent factors, 11
5-methyltetrahydrofolate (5-MTHF), 147
fluorescence resonance energy transfer (FRET), 176
fluorescence in-situ hybridisation (FISH),
        43, 69, 75

G

gall stones, 159
gastrointestinal symptoms, 147
gastrointestinal tract (GIT), 143
genetics
        beta thalassaemia, 120
        essential thrombocytosis, 49–50
        G6PD, 160–161
        haemophilia A, 7–8
        hereditary spherocytosis, 165
        testing, 8
germinal centre B-cell-like (GCB), 69
glomerular basement membrane (GBM), 103

glucose-6-phosphate dehydrogenase (G6PD)
   biliary pancreatitis, 159
   bite cells, *160*
   clinical progress, 159
   clinical scenario, 159
   diagnosis, 161
   gall stones, 159
   genetics, 160–161
   haematological effects, 161
   hemighosts, *160*
   laboratory reports, 159
   management, 162
   oxidative haemolysis in, **161**
   physiology, 159–160
   questions, 159
glycosylphosphatidylinositol (GPI), 138
graft-versus-host disease (GVHD), 31
granulocyte colony-stimulating factor (G-CSF), 41
gray zone lymphoma, 98

H

haematological malignancies, 185
haematopoietic stem cell (HSC), 69
haematopoietic stem cell transplantation (HSCT), 31, 37,
      56, 106
haemoglobin H (HbH) disease
   clinical presentations, 125
   clinical progress, 123
   clinical scenario, 123
   differential diagnosis, 125
   laboratory findings, 125
   laboratory reports, 123
   malaise, 123
   management, 126
   pathogenesis, 124–125
   peripheral blood smear, *124*
   questions, 123
   thalassaemia syndromes, 124
haemolytic anaemia, 73
haemolytic uraemic syndrome (HUS), 178
haemophagocytic lymphohistiocytosis (HLH)
   bone marrow aspirate, *197*
   clinical presentation, 198
   clinical progress, 196
   clinical scenario, 196
   diagnosis, 198, **199**
   fever and myalgia, 196
   laboratory reports, 196
   pathophysiology, 198
   questions, 197
   treatment, 199
haemophilia A
   clinical scenario, 7
   coagulation pathways, *8*
   dcfinition, 7
   differential diagnosis, 9
   genetics, 7–8
   genetic testing, 8
   joint swelling, 7
   laboratory reports, 7
   management, 9–10
   questions, 7
hairy cell leukaemia (HCL)

clinical characteristics, 82
clinical progress, 80
clinical scenario, 80
laboratory reports, 80
pathological characteristics, 81–82
in peripheral blood, *81*
questions, 80
renal stone, 80
treatment, 82
variant, 82
HbH disease, *see* haemoglobin H (HbH) disease
HCL variant (HCLv), 82
Helicobacter pylori, 143, 146
HELLP syndrome, 175
hepatitis B
   disseminated intravascular coagulopathy (DIC), 21
   myelodysplastic syndrome (MDS), 39
hepatitis C virus (HCV), 119
hereditary macrothrombocytopenia
   blood film, *188*
   cataract, 187
   clinical progress, 187
   clinical relevance, 189
   clinical scenario, 187
   definition, 187–188
   diagnosis, 189
   laboratory reports, 187
   questions, 187
hereditary spherocytosis (HS)
   clinical scenario, 163
   definition, 163
   diagnoses, 164
   genetics, 165
   laboratory reports, 163
   management, 165
   polychromasia, *164*
   questions, 163
   spherocytosis, *164*
   vomiting and diarrhoea, 163
HES, *see* hypereosinophilic syndrome (HES)
high-performanceliquid chromatography (HPLC),
      121, 127
Hodgkin lymphoma
   allergic rhinitis, 96
   clinical progress, 96–97
   clinical scenario, 96
   differential diagnoses, 98
   eczema, 96
   histological features, *97*
   questions, 96
   treatment and prognosis, 98–99
HSC, *see* haematopoietic stem cell (HSC)
HSCT, *see* haematopoietic stem cell transplantation
      (HSCT)
human immunodeficiency virus (HIV) infection, 209
HUS, *see* haemolytic uraemic syndrome (HUS)
hydroxyurea, 129
hypereosinophilic syndrome (HES)
   bone marrow aspirate, *201*
   clinical presentation, 202
   clinical progress, 200
   clinical scenario, 200
   laboratory reports, 200
   management, 202–203

peripheral blood smear, *201*
questions, 200
vomiting and diarrhoea, 200
hypergammaglobulinaemia, *see* lymphadenopathy
hyperlipidaemia
    acute myeloid leukaemia II, 35
    amyloidosis, 103
    Castleman disease, 193
    POEMS syndrome, 113
hyperviscosity, 72–73
hypoplastic MDS (hMDS), 139

I

idiopathic hypereosinophilia, 202
IgG4–related diseases, 208
immune thrombocytopenia (ITP)
    clinical features, 183–184
    clinical progress, 183
    diagnosis, 185
    easy bruising, 183
    laboratory reports, 183
    management, 185–186
    pathogenesis, *184*, 184–185
    questions, 183
immunoglobulin G4–related disease (IgG4–RD)
    clinical scenario, 204
    definition, 204–205
    differential diagnoses, 206
    investigations, 205–206
    laboratory reports, 204
    lymphocytes, *205*
    plasma cells, *205*
    questions, 204
    rheumatoid arthritis, 204
    treatment, 206
immunohistochemistry (IHC), 69
immunosuppression, 176
implantable cardioverter defibrillator (ICD), 106
infection–associated HUS, 179
International Prognostic Index (IPI), 70
International Prognostic Scoring System (IPSS), 56
International Staging System (ISS), 110
iron deficiency anaemia (IDA)
    causes, 143
    clinical scenario, 141
    haemoglobin, *142*
    investigations, 143–144
    iron metabolism, 141–142
    laboratory results, 141
    questions, 141
    shortness of breath, 141
    symptoms, 143
    treatment, 144
iron metabolism, 141–142
ischaemic stroke, 129
isolated APTT prolongation
    acquired Factor VIII inhibitor, 16
    clinical scenario, 14
    clinical progress, 14
    definition, 14–16
    laboratory reports, 14
    questions, 14
    treatment, 16–17

J

joint swelling, *see* haemophilia A

L

lactate dehydrogenase (LDH), 55
langerhans cell histiocytosis (LCH)
    asthma, 61
    cell of origin in, *63*
    clinical presentation, 62
    clinical scenario, 61
    cutaneous presentation, 62
    definition, 61
    hepatic involvement, 62
    investigations, 62–64
    molecular pathogenesis, 62
    pulmonary presentation, 62
    questions, 61
    skeletal involvement, 62
    treatment, 64
langerhans cells (LCs), 61
large granular lymphocyte leukaemia (LGLL), 137
leg ulcers, 130
localised amyloidosis, 105
low molecular weight heparin (LMWH), 27
lupus anticoagulant (LA), 18
lymphadenopathy, 75
    causes, 207–208
    clinical progress, 209
    clinical scenario, 207
    HIV infection, 209
    investigations, 209
    laboratory reports, 207
    PET/CT scan, *208*
    questions, 207
    weight loss, 207
lymphocyte predominant (LP), 97
lymphocyte-varianthypereosinophilia, 202
lymphoplasmacytic lymphoma (LPL), 73
lymphoproliferative diseases, 201

M

magnetic resonance imaging (MRI), 61
MAHA, *see* microangiopathic haemolytic anaemia
    (MAHA)
marrow fibrosis, 56
Mayo Stratification of Myeloma and Risk-Adapted
    Therapy (mSMART), 110
MCM, *see* methylmalonyl-CoA mutase (MCM)
MDS, *see* myelodysplastic syndrome (MDS)
methaemoglobinaemia
    causes of, 133
    clinical presentation, 133–134
    clinical progress, 131
    clinical scenario, 131
    dermatitis herpetiformis, 131
    laboratory reports, 131–132
    methylene blue, *132*
    oxygen transfer, 132–133
    pulse oximetry in, 133
    questions, 131
    saturation gap, 133

treatment, 134
methicillin-sensitive *Staphylococcus aureus* (MSSA), 94, 210
methionine synthase (MS), 147
methylcobalamin, 147
methylmalonyl-CoA mutase (MCM), 147
MF, *see* mycosis fungoides (MF)
microangiopathic haemolytic anaemia (MAHA), 175
minimal (measurable) residual disease (MRD) monitoring, 33, *45*
monoclonal gammopathy of unknown significance (MGUS), 110
MPN, *see* myeloproliferative neoplasm (MPN)
MSSA, *see* methicillin-sensitive *Staphylococcus aureus* (MSSA)
mucosal associated lymphoid tissue (MALT), 206
multicentric(MCD), 194
multicentric Castleman disease, 208
multiple myeloma (MM)
    abnormal plasma cells, 109
    bone marrow, *108*
    clinical features, 110
    clinical scenario, 107
    definition, 109
    investigations, 110
    laboratory reports, 107
    lytic lesions, *109*
    management, 111–112
    organ damage, 109
    paraproteins, 109
    pathogenesis, 110
    prognostication, 110–111
    progress, 107–108
    questions, 107
    treatment, 108–109, **111**
multiplex ligation-dependent probe amplification (MLPA), 8
Mycobacterium haemophilum, 94
mycosis fungoides (MF)
    clinical presentation, 90
    clinical scenario, 90
    definition, 90
    erythematous rash, 90
    histological features of, *91*
    investigations, 91
    PET/CT scan, 90
    prognosis, 91
    questions, 90
    treatment, 91–92
myelodysplastic syndrome (MDS), 33, 58
    clinical scenario, 39
    definition, 40–41
    differential diagnosis, 41
    hepatitis B, 39
    high-risk, 41
    hypolobated and hypogranular neutrophil, *40*
    laboratory reports, 39
    low-risk, 41
    pathogenesis, 41
    progress, 39, 40
    questions, 39
    treatment, 41
myeloid neoplasm with germline predisposition
    anaemia, 58
    classification of, **59**
    clinical scenario, 58
    definition, 58–60
    investigations, 58
    patient progress, 58
    pedigree of, *59*
    questions, 58
    RUNX1 mutation, 60
myeloproliferative neoplasm (MPN), 33, 55

N

NK/T-cell lymphoma
    clinical progress, 87
    clinical scenario, 87
    clinical subtypes of, 87–88
    definition, 87
    nasal biopsy, *88*
    questions, 87
nephropathy, 130
nerve conduction velocity (NCV), 113
neurological defects, 147
neuropsychiatric defects, 147
neutrophil extracellular traps (NETs), 25
next generation sequencing (NGS), 8, 39, 48
nicotinamide adenine dinucleotide phosphate (NADP), 159
NK cell leukaemia, 88
non-Hodgkin lymphoma (NHL), 90
nonimmune microangiopathic haemolytic anaemia, 178
non-nasal type lymphoma, 88
non-neoplastic inflammatory cells, 96
non-transfusion-dependent thalassaemia (NTDT), 121, 124

O

obinutuzumab and bendamustine (OB), 210
oral L-glutamine, 129

P

paraneoplastic pemphigus (PNP)
    balanitis, 210
    clinical features of, *211*
    clinical progress, 210
    clinical scenario, 210
    definition, 212
    laboratory reports, 210
    pathogenesis, 212
    questions, 210
    treatment, 212–213
paravalvular leak
    cardiac prosthesis-related haemolytic anaemia, 167
    clinical progress, 166
    clinical scenario, 166
    laboratory reports, 166
    microangiopathic change, *167*
    questions, 166
    rheumatic heart disease, 166
paroxysmal cold haemoglobinuria (PCH), 155
paroxysmal nocturnal haemoglobinuria (PNH), 137, 143, 166
    clinical manifestations, 171
    clinical progress, 169–170

clinical scenario, 169
diagnosis, 171
easy bruising, 169
haematological response, *170*
laboratory reports, 169
pathogenesis, 170–171
questions, 169
treatment, 171–172
PE, *see* pulmonary embolism (PE)
pentose phosphate pathway (PPP), 159
percutaneous coronary intervention (PCI), 43
Periodic Schiff-Methenamine Silver (PASM), 103
peripheral neuropathy, 72
pernicious anaemia (PA), 148–149
Philadelphia chromosome (Ph)–positive acute
     lymphoblastic leukaemia (ALL)
    blood smear, *84*
    bone pain and fever, 83
    clinical scenario, 83
    laboratory reports, 83
    patient progress, 83
    precursor B-cell ALL, 85
    questions, 83
    treatment, 85
phosphoinositide 3-kinase (PI3k), 78
plasmapheresis, 176
plasminogen activator inhibitor-1 (PAI-1), 22
PNP, *see* paraneoplastic pemphigus (PNP)
POEMS syndrome
    clinical scenario, 113
    definition, 113–115
    diagnostic criteria, **115**
    hyperlipidaemia, 113
    laboratory reports, 113
    osteosclerotic focus, *114*
    patient progress, 115
    questions, 113
    treatment, 116
polycythaemia vera (PV)
    clinical features, 52
    clinical progress, 51
    clinical scenario, 51
    complications, 53
    laboratory reports in 2013, 51
    laboratory reports in 2021, 51–52
    management plan, 53
    palpable spleen tip, 51
    patients with localised disease, 116
    patients with systemic disease, 116
    peripheral blood smear of, *52*
    prognosis, 53
    questions, 51
positron emission tomography/computed tomography
    (PET/CT), 67, *68*, *114*, 196, *208*
precursor B-cell ALL, 85
priapism, 130
primary bone marrow disorder, 201
primary mediastinal B-cell lymphoma (PMBCL), 98
primary myelofibrosis (PMF)
    anaemia, 56
    atrial flutter, 54
    clinical presentation, 54–55
    clinical progress, 54
    clinical scenario, 54

constitutional symptoms, 56
diagnosis, 55–56
laboratory reports, 54
prognostication, 56
questions, 54
splenomegaly, 56
treatment, 56
trephine biopsy, *55*
prolonged APTT, 5
prolonged PT
    acquired Factor V inhibitor, 18–19
    DIC, 18–19, 22
    Factor VII deficiency, 11
prothrombin time (PT)
    acquired Factor V (FV) inhibitor, 18–19
    VWD, 5
pulmonary embolism (PE), 24
pulmonary hypertension, 130
pulse oximetry, 133

R

receptor activator of NFκB ligand (RANKL), 112
recombinant activated factor VIIa (rFVIIa), 9
red cell transfusion, 56
retinopathy, 130
revised ISS, 110
rheumatoid arthritis (RA), 204
ristocetin-induced platelet aggregation (RIPA), 3
rituximab, 176, 195
rituximab, cyclophosphamide, hydroxydaunorubicin,
    oncovin and prednisolone (R-CHOP), 69
RUNX1 mutation, 60

S

S-adenosylmethionine (SAM), 147
scattered large mononuclear Hodgkin cells, 96
serum amyloid A (SAA), 105
serum protein electrophoresis (SPEP), 113
severe acute respiratory syndrome coronavirus 2
    (SARS-CoV-2), 153
severe haemophilia A, *see* haemophilia A
sickle cell disease (SCD)
    acute sickling crises, 129–130
    bilateral lower limb swelling, 127
    chronic sickle cell diseases, 130
    clinical progress, 127
    clinical scenario, 127
    definition, 129
    laboratory reports, 127
    management, 129
    pathogenesis, 129
    prevention, 129
    questions, 127
    red cells, *128*
small lymphocytic lymphoma (SLL), 77
splenectomy, 176
systemic lupus erythematosus (SLE), 183

T

tartrate-resistant acid phosphatase (TRAP), 82
T-cell prolymphocytic leukaemia (T-PLL)

clinical progress, 93–94
clinical scenario, 93
definition, 94
hepatitis, 93
laboratory reports, 93
management, 94–95
peripheral blood, *94*
questions, 93
T-cell receptor (TCR), 204
thalassaemia syndromes, 124
therapy-related AML (t-AML), 33
thrombocytopenia, 21, 178
thrombopoietin mimetics, 186
thrombotic microangiopathy (TMA), 175
  during pregnancy, 178
thrombotic thrombocytopenic purpura (TTP), 21
  anaemia, 173
  causes, 175–176
  clinical features, 175
  clinical progress, 173
  clinical scenario, 173
  expressive dysphasia, 173
  investigations, 176
  laboratory reports, 173
  management, 176
  pathogenesis, 175
  questions, 173
  schistocytes, *174*
  TMA, 175
thrombosis, 22
tissue plasminogen activator (t-PA), 22
total iron–binding capacity (TIBC), 143
transferrin receptors (TFR), 141, 142
transfusion-dependent thalassaemia (TDT), 121, 124
type 1 Von Willebrand disease (VWD), 4
type 2 Von Willebrand disease (VWD), 4
type 3 Von Willebrand disease (VWD), 5
tyrosine kinase inhibitor (TKI), 85
  first generation, 46
  fourth generation, 46
  second generation, 46
  third generation, 46

U

unicentric (UCD), 193, 194
Upshaw–Schulman syndrome, 175

V

variable region of immunoglobulin gene heavy chain (IGHV), 77
vascular endothelial growth factor (VEGF), 113
venous thromboembolism (VTE)
  causes of, **26**
  clinical progress, 24
  clinical scenario, 24
  colonic polyps and diverticulosis, 24
  complications, 28
  CT, 24
  diagnosis, 27
  duration of treatment, 28

  laboratory reports, 24
  pathogenesis, 24–25
  pathogenesis of, *26*
  questions, 24
  radiological diagnosis, 27
  risk factors, 25–27
  treatment, 27–28
  tumour masses, *25*
vitamin B12 deficiency anaemia
  absorption, 147
  bone marrow features, 148
  causes, 148
  cellular function, 147
  clinical manifestations, 147
  clinical progress, 145
  clinical scenario, 145
  diabetes, 145
  hypertension, 145
  laboratory features, 147–148
  laboratory reports, 145
  laboratory tests, 145–146
  megaloblastic anaemia, *146*
  pernicious anaemia, 148–149
  questions, 145
  sources of, *146*
  treatment, 149
Von Willebrand disease (VWD), 4–5
Von Willebrand factor (VWF)
  clinical progress, 3–4
  clinical scenario, 3
  definition, 4–5
  diagnosis of, 5
  differential diagnosis of, 5
  easy bruising, 3
  laboratory reports, 3
  management, 5–6
  multimeric study, *4*
  questions, 3
voxelotor, 129

W

Waldenström macroglobulinaemia (WM)
  bone marrow infiltration, *72*
  clinical manifestations, 72–73
  clinical progress, 71
  clinical scenario, 71
  definition, 71
  diagnosis, 73
  fever and malaise, 71
  management, 73
  questions, 71
warm-type autoimmune haemolytic anaemia
  clinical scenario, 153
  diagnosis, 153
  differential diagnoses, 154–155
  hypertension and diabetes, 153
  laboratory reports, 153
  management, 155
  pathogenesis, 154
  polychromasia and spherocytosis, *154*
  questions, 153